Strong & Fit After 40

WOMEN'S HEALTH

Strong & Fit After 40

4 Weeks to Lifelong Fitness at Home

Ashley Nicole, CPT, and the editors of *Women's Health*

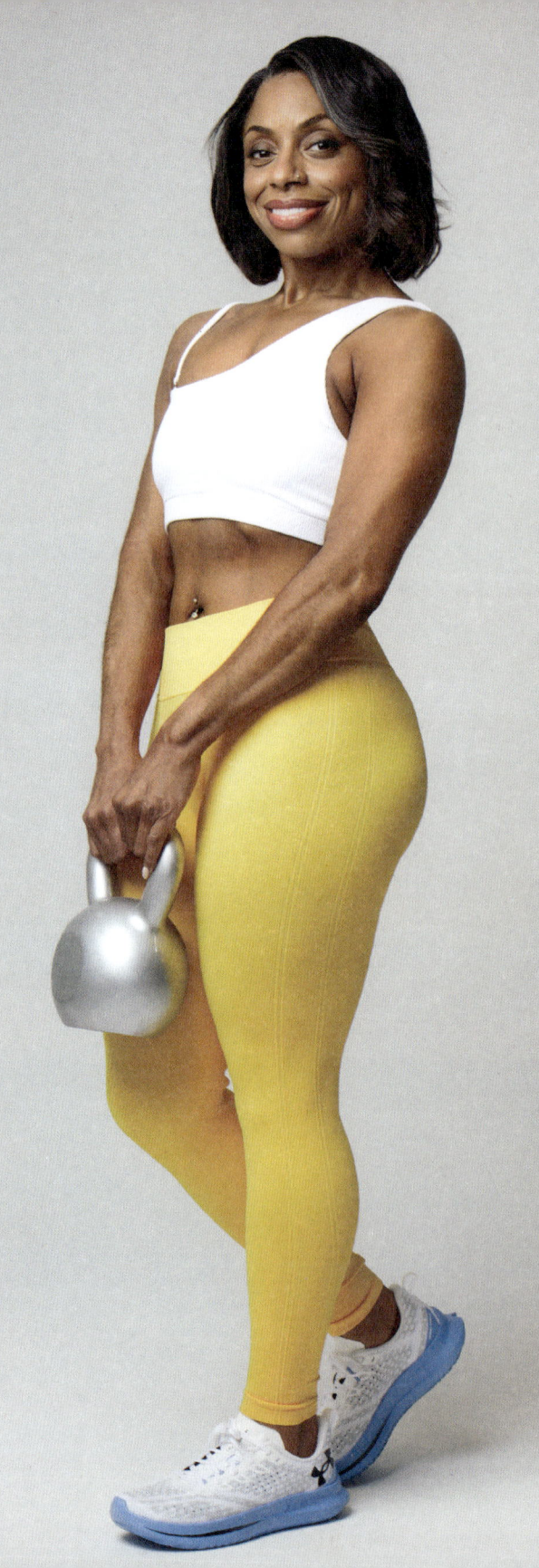

Contents

▶ **Introduction**

The Simple Way to Get Fitter Than Ever at 40+ **6**

▶ **Chapter 1**

How Your Body Changes After 40 and What to Do About It **8**

▶ **Chapter 2**

The Key to Staying Strong as You Age **16**

▶ **Chapter 3**

The 28-Day Plan **28**
- Week 1 **35**
- Week 2 **47**
- Week 3 **61**
- Week 4 **75**

▶ **Chapter 4**

Exercise Guide **88**
- Upper Body **90**
  - Single Single Double Biceps Curl **91**
  - Chest Fly **92**
  - Rear Delt Fly **93**
  - Triceps Kickback **94**
  - Bridge Chest Press **95**
  - Shuffle Punch **96**
  - Incline Pushup **97**
  - Alternating Front and Lateral Raise **98**
  - Isometric Lateral Raise **99**
- Lower Body **100**
  - Banded Glute Bridge **101**
  - Clamshell **102**
  - Staggered-Stance Deadlift **103**
  - Figure Four to Twist **104**
  - Reverse Lunge **105**
  - Football Shuffle **106**
  - Banded Lateral Step-Out Squat **107**
  - Dumbbell Sumo Squat **108**
  - Jump Squat **109**
  - Lying Hip Flexor Stretch **110**
- Core **111**
  - 90/90 Tap **112**
  - Deadbug **113**
  - Loaded Deadbug **114**
  - Farmer's Carry **115**
  - Inchworm Shoulder Tap **116**
  - Knee Drive **117**
  - Marching Glute Bridge **118**
  - Mountain Climber **119**
  - Plank Walkout **120**
  - Reverse Crunch **121**
  - Scissor Kick **122**
  - Superman **123**
  - T-Spine Rotation **124**
  - Thread the Needle **125**
  - V-Up **126**
  - Warrior One Row **127**
- Total Body **128**
  - Child's Pose **129**
  - Good Morning **130**
  - Jumping Jack **131**
  - Modified Burpee **132**
  - Dead Clean **133**
  - Curtsy Lunge With Biceps Curl **134**
  - Side Lunge and Row **135**
  - Deadlift and Row **136**
  - Squat and Snatch **137**
  - Squat to Overhead Press **138**
  - Squat to Single-Arm Overhead Press **139**

INTRODUCTION

The Simple Way to Get Fitter Than Ever at 40+

I WANT TO START OFF BY GIVING YOU ONE short-and-sweet message: Congratulations!

If you're reading this book, I'm guessing you've already made it to that amazing four-decade milestone and have decided to take another step toward living your healthiest, happiest life. That deserves a moment of celebration.

And if you're like me and so many women over 40, you've no doubt encountered some hurdles along the path to wellness. Maybe you're dealing with hormonal changes and the symptoms that come with them (hello, hot flashes, mood swings, and insomnia!), a slower metabolism, low energy, and weakened muscles or muscle loss. Perhaps you're contending with the cumulative effects of previous injuries or a sedentary life, like weight gain and joint pain. As a trainer in her 40s with rheumatoid arthritis, I've had to face the added challenge of working through joint pain, stiffness, and inflammation. I know what it's like to deal with physical obstacles—and rise above them (it's why I named my business RA Warrior Fitness to begin with). Whatever your current situation, I'm here to tell you it's not only possible to make your 40s and beyond your fittest years yet, but that it can also be done with one simple solution: strength training.

Strength training can supercharge so many aspects of your health. The more muscle you have, the better equipped your body is to combat the physical changes that come with aging and hormonal shifts. Muscle stabilizes your joints to improve mobility, boosts metabolism to aid in weight management, and supports bone density to prevent osteoporosis (the weakening of bones that leads to breakage). In short, building and maintaining muscle promotes longevity.

And it's truly easier than ever to enjoy these benefits. I've spent years finding real-life solutions to help women over 40 get fit, and now I'm sharing those secrets with you in my new 28-day workout plan. It's designed to make prioritizing your wellness simple. This program is fast (every workout is 30 minutes or less), at-home-friendly (you just need a few pieces of equipment), and efficient (you'll target multiple muscles at once for maximum benefit). And—best of all—it's incredibly fun. Give it just one day and I know you'll add it to your list of reasons to celebrate.

So rise up, warriors, and let's get to work!

ASHLEY NICOLE, CPT, a.k.a. Coach Ash

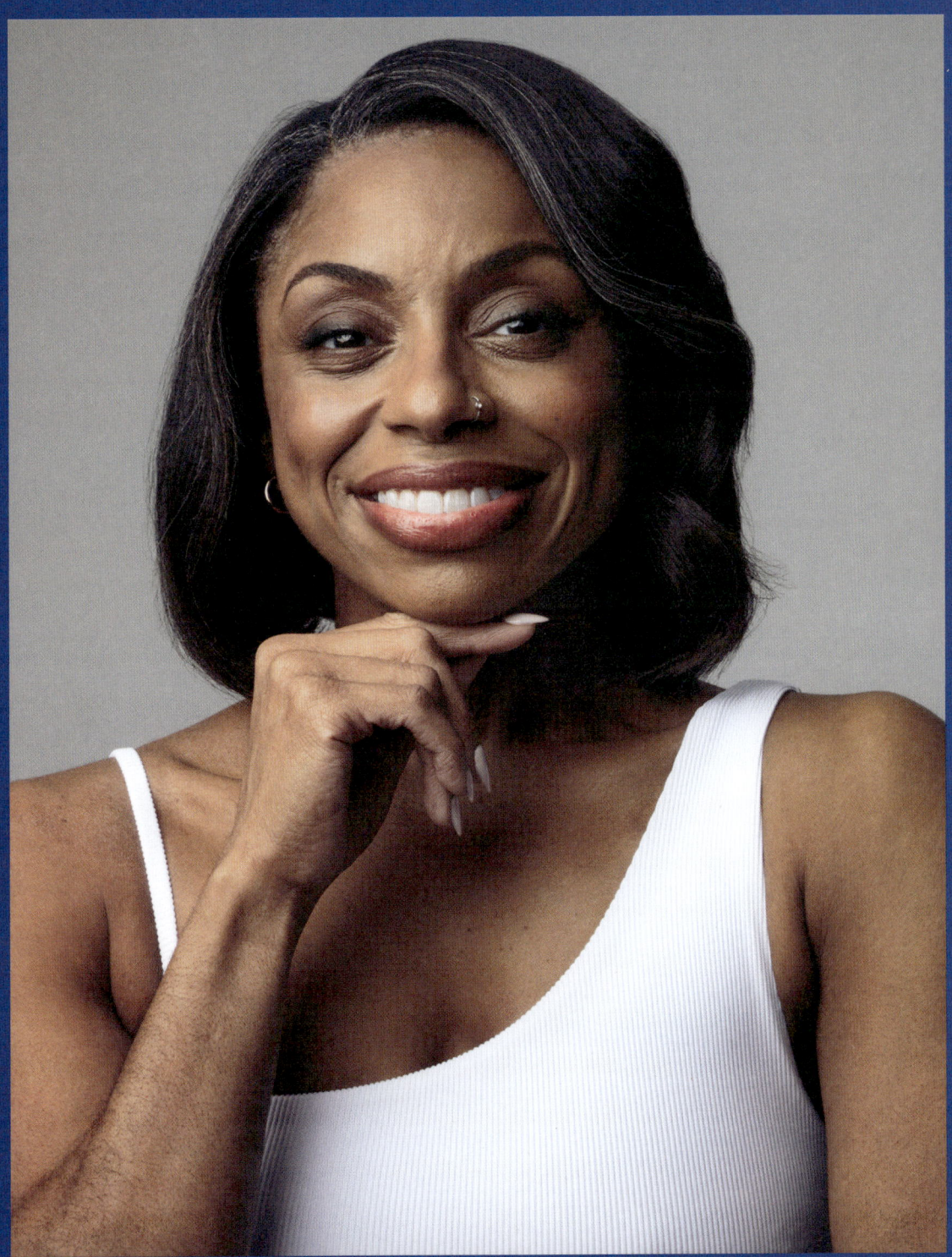

CHAPTER 1

How Your Body Changes After 40 and What to Do About It

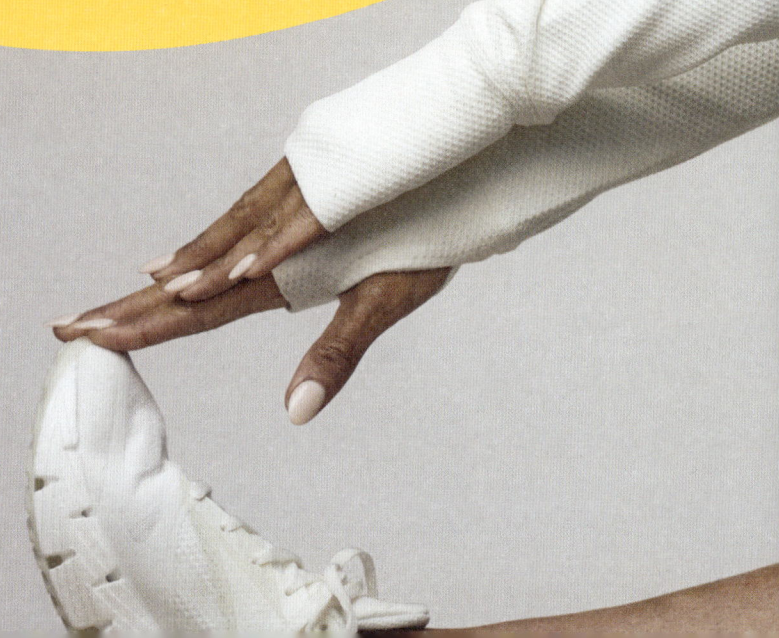

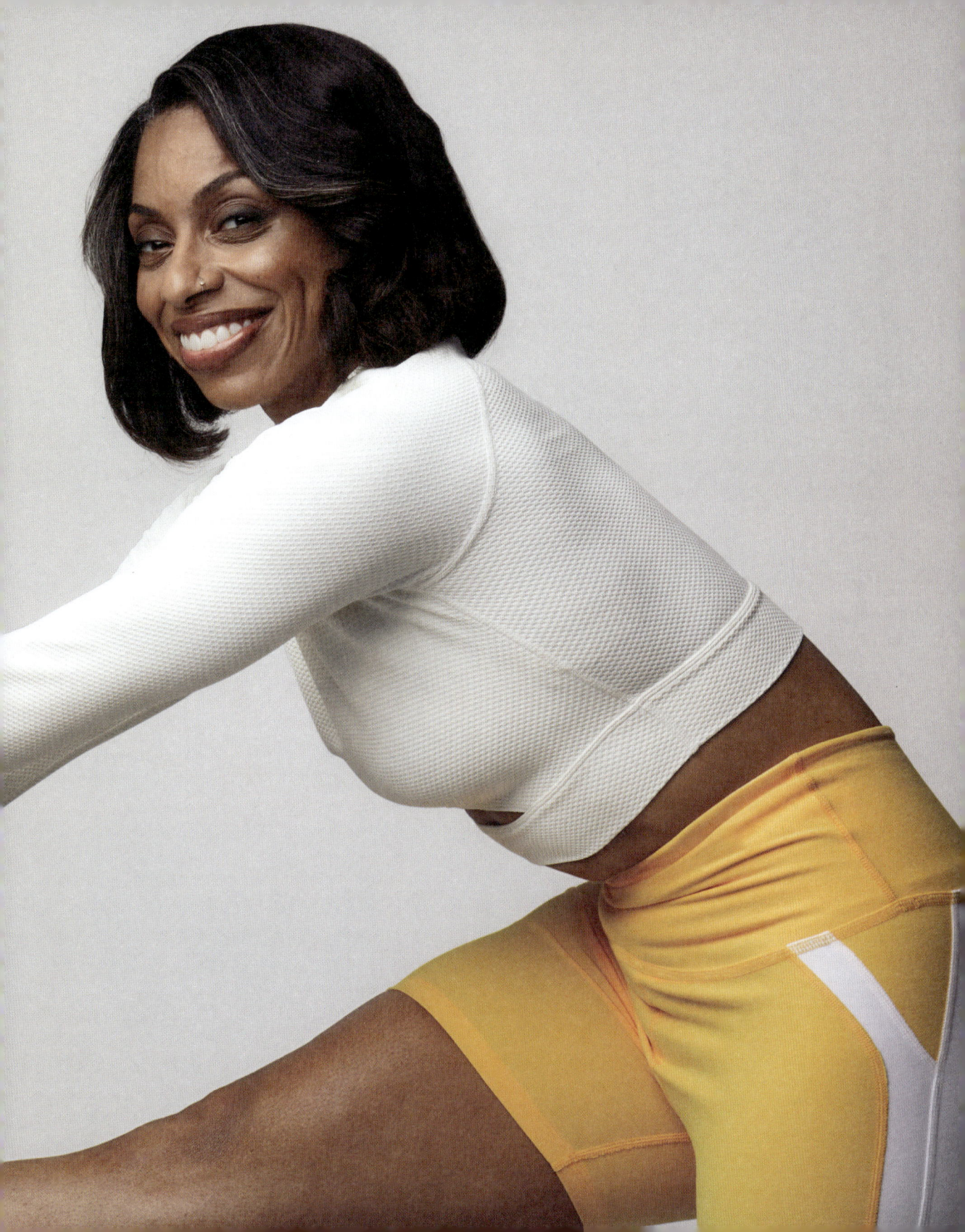

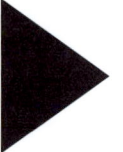 **Getting older comes with plenty of positives: wisdom from years of life experiences, a greater appreciation for the little things, and tons of unforgettable memories, to name a few.**

But each decade of your life can also bring specific changes to your health, like decreased mobility and flexibility, muscle loss, weakened joints and bones, slower metabolism, and a whole host of illnesses like high blood pressure, heart disease, and chronic pain.

While some parts of aging are unavoidable, many of the problems we associate with getting older can actually be offset by something completely within your control: how much you move. In study after study, regular workouts have been proven to insulate you from heart disease, cancer, Alzheimer's, stroke, and diabetes. Exercise lowers blood pressure, reduces body fat, raises "good" cholesterol, lowers "bad" cholesterol, improves blood flow, keeps intestines and the colon healthy, and regulates key hormones. In other words, regular sweat sessions can help rewind the clock on aging.

Even better? You can supercharge those positive effects of exercise if you adjust your routine to wherever you are at in life (and the unique fitness hurdles that can accompany it). Here's a decade-by-decade breakdown of how to adapt your fitness habits to feel your best at every age.

In Your 40s
The Busy Decade

The Challenge:

LACK OF TIME FOR EXERCISE

This may be your busiest decade yet—and, as a result, you might put other important parts of your life ahead of physical activity. But without regular exercise, strength and cardiovascular fitness can begin to decline rapidly.

What You Can Do:

MAKE WORKOUTS SHORTER BUT MORE EFFECTIVE

Researchers have found that brief but physically challenging exercise sessions can improve your health just as much as longer sessions can. In a three-month study at McMaster University in Canada, one group of participants rode a stationary bicycle at a steady, moderate pace for 45 minutes three times a week. Another group cycled for seven minutes three days a week, alternating pedaling as fast as possible for 20 seconds with slowing down to an easy, relaxed pace for two minutes.

At the end of the experiment, the people in the short-workout group improved their markers of cardio fitness and insulin sensitivity just as much as the people who cycled for 45 minutes. You can mimic the brief-but-intense style—you know it as high-intensity interval training (HIIT)—with almost any type of cardio exercise.

SNEAK MOVEMENT IN ALL DAY

Every little bit of physical activity counts. Think about taking the long way to your favorite coffee shop. Or put that smart watch to work by setting a reminder to get up and move every hour. "Whether it's taking the stairs instead of the elevator, parking further away to add a few extra steps, or doing a quick set of squats while waiting for your coffee to brew, these small actions can add up to significant health benefits over time," says Coach Ash. Bonus: Adding extra bursts of activity to your day throughout the 28-day plan in this book can boost your results even more.

INCREASE STRENGTH

Strength training is always a good idea, but it's essential in your 40s and beyond as you slowly lose muscle mass. Adding more strength exercises to your fitness routine will help build more muscle and fortify the systems in your body that help with mobility, injury prevention, and endurance. However, when you're in your busiest decade yet, it can be a struggle to fit in a comprehensive workout.

Instead of packing your routine with separate exercises for every body part, save time by doing moves that hit multiple muscles at once.

QUICK WAYS TO ADD MOVEMENT THROUGHOUT YOUR DAY

WHEN YOU'RE WORKING:

- Set your alarm every half hour to remind you to take a two- to three-minute lap around your office.
- Do some desk stretches every two hours.
- Take the stairs instead of the elevator.

WHILE RUNNING ERRANDS:

- Instead of just standing in line at the grocery, try practicing pelvic lifts. Shift your weight back to your heels, then push your right hip toward the floor to lift your left foot slightly off the ground. Switch sides and repeat.
- Do shoulder rolls as you're waiting for your turn at the bank.

ON BUSY DAYS:

- Take 15 minutes to perform hip-opening yoga moves (try pigeon pose or happy baby).
- Remember to get up and get a glass of water as often as possible so you move and stay hydrated at the same time.

OVER THE WEEKEND:

- Go for a jog or longer yoga sweat session.
- Run around with or lift your kids at the playground.
- Garden on your hands and knees.

When programmed correctly, these moves—known as compound exercises—not only maximize your time and effort on the mat, but also improve daily functions. (Squats, for example, strengthen basically every muscle in your lower body, while reinforcing your ability to sit and stand with ease.) Luckily, the right strength training program, like the one in this book, can combat muscle loss and help improve everyday movement, so you feel stronger than ever in no time.

In Your 50s
The Decade of Change

The Challenge:

ESTROGEN DECLINE
When estrogen declines during perimenopause and menopause, your muscles begin to lose their size and strength, says Coach Ash. Plus, your body's ability to metabolize blood sugar decreases, and fat accumulates more easily around your middle. The change even goes one layer deeper, causing an imbalance in skeletal turnover that exacerbates decreases in bone density.

What You Can Do:

FIND AN ACTIVITY YOU LOVE AND MAKE IT ROUTINE
Can a consistent fitness program eliminate the negative effects of waning estrogen? More and more studies are showing promising results. When your body stops producing estrogen, it can lead to a lot of health issues, the most common of which are hot flashes and night sweats that negatively impact your sleep, which is crucial for recovery. But a German study that lasted three years showed that early postmenopausal women who did a combination of aerobic and strength-training exercises four days a week experienced fewer bouts with insomnia compared to the sedentary participants. They also maintained bone mass, lost 2 percent body fat and an inch off their midsection, and reduced cholesterol by 5 percent.

Incorporating any workout will help alleviate a lot of the symptoms that come with hormonal changes and your 50s is the ideal time to create an exercise schedule you can stick with. The trick is finding an activity that excites you and is so much fun that you'd hate to miss it. Then make sure that you're increasing the intensity week-by-week (like we'll do in this plan) so you can get stronger.

PUSH YOURSELF HARDER
Research shows that bouts of vigorous exercise deliver the greatest benefits and can be particularly helpful with menopausal challenges like hot flashes, insomnia, and weight gain. In a study in the *Journal of Physiology*, women going through menopause who performed moderately intense workouts kept their hot flashes to a minimum as opposed to the control group who did not exercise.

Better yet, you can get the perks of dialing up the intensity whether you do cardio or strength training. In other studies, high-intensity cardio routines helped overweight women reduce fat around their midsection better than slow and steady workouts did. To get the same cardiovascular benefits from your strength workout, increase your effort by using

THE MERIT OF MULTI-TASKING

Stay motivated by pairing workouts with an activity you look forward to, like listening to a podcast. Your brain gets a hit of pleasure, which you'll then associate with exercise.

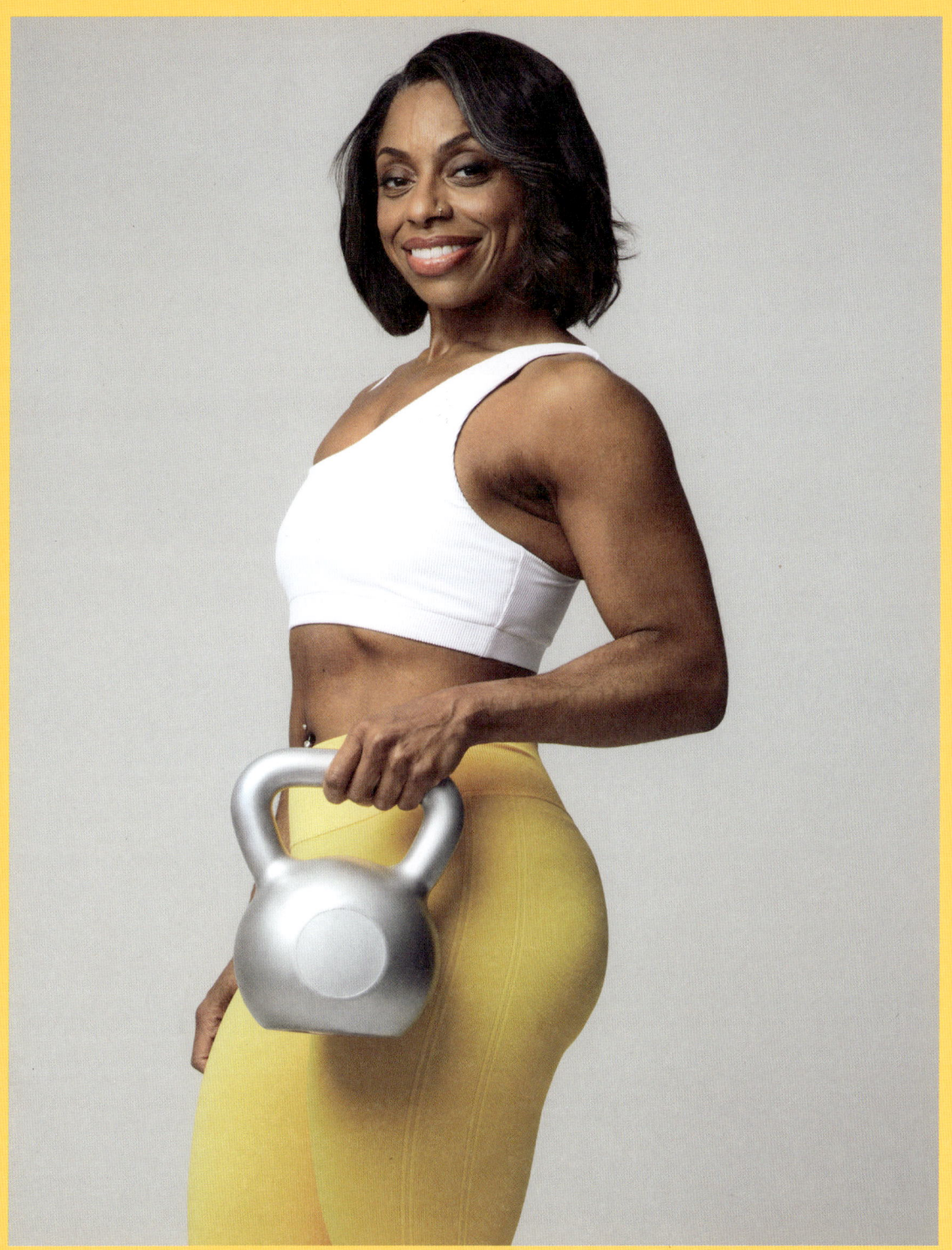

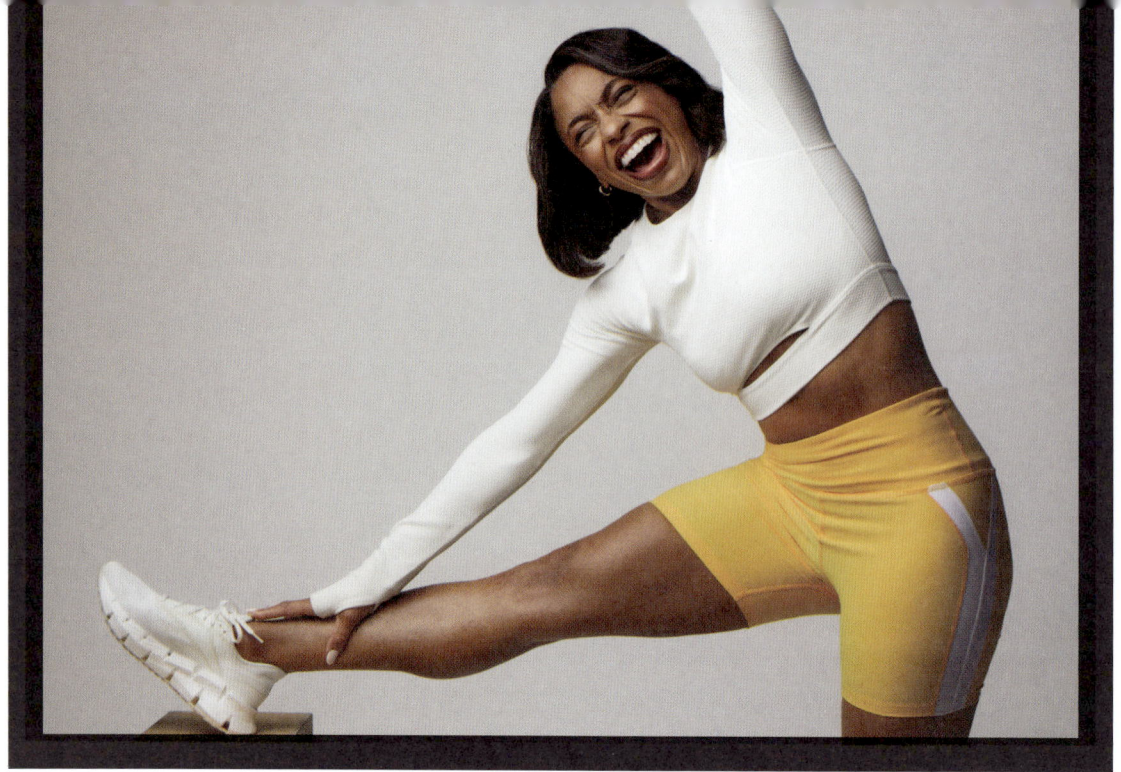

heavier weights and higher reps each week (which you'll do in the 28-day plan). This method, known as progressive overload, can help reduce body fat, extend your post-workout burn, improve sleep habits, build muscle, and make you stronger, while also boosting your balance and posture and cutting your injury risk.

TRY BONE-BOOSTING EXERCISES
Your body is constantly breaking down and rebuilding bone (a process known as bone remodeling), but as your estrogen levels dip, you begin to lose more bone than you make. What's more, the bones you already have may weaken, putting you at greater risk for fractures. But estrogen isn't the only thing that matters when it comes to strong, healthy bones. The right type of exercise can actually help build back what you've lost.

Scientists think that moderate impact on your bones—the kind that comes from exercises like hiking, dancing, playing tennis, and lifting weights—is key to triggering your skeleton to lay down more minerals. With the right routine, like the one programmed in this book, you can increase bone density by as much as 2 percent a year.

In Your 60s
The Stay-Strong Decade

The Challenge:

MUSCLE LOSS
Sarcopenia, or muscle loss, is a natural part of the aging process. You can lose as much as 3 to 5 percent of your muscle mass each decade if you're not regularly active. That steady muscle drain will start catching up with you, making it harder to get up from sitting on the floor or lift a heavy bag of groceries.

What You Can Do:

BUILD MUSCLE
The muscles you build help you stay strong and insulate your body from injury. And you can do this at any age in a relatively short time. In fact, it took only 10 weeks for a group of people in their 60s to increase their leg strength by 42 percent, according to a study in the *Journal of Strength and Conditioning Research*. This 28-day strength training

program is designed with effective workouts you can do in less than 30 minutes so you can build muscle and strength even in as little as one month.

DO "FUNCTIONAL EXERCISES"

These are moves that mimic the way you use your body in daily life, such as squatting, bending down, lifting, and reaching. Stronger hips and glutes allow you to walk longer, climb stairs better, and reduce your chances of falling, says Breena Maggio, director of a restorative exercise studio in Ventura, California. "Stronger butt muscles can also mean a healthier pelvic floor, helpful for women who experience incontinence," she adds.

Also, bodyweight movements prepare your muscles for the ways they'll be used every day, whether it's sitting properly in a chair or going up and down staircases and hills. They'll improve your reaction time to catch yourself when you trip and develop every muscle in your body to its full potential. By focusing on movements instead of specific muscle groups, you improve your entire neuromuscular system, not just your muscles, and advance your overall body awareness and coordination.

GET CREATIVE WITH CARDIO

Just like in every decade prior, you still need cardiovascular exercise that elevates your heart rate and puts a smile on your face. But you don't have to stick to the same exact cardio workout forever. Look for opportunities to refresh your routine. If you love walking, try mixing up your existing regimen by taking a new route, listening to an audiobook, or inviting a friend to join. Or give a new type of cardio a go and sign up for that dance class you've been meaning to take! Just be sure to schedule these sessions for days when you aren't doing another type of exercise that works the same body parts.

Through Every Decade

The Challenge:

POOR BALANCE

You might think you only need to work on your balance for a yoga session, but stability is important to your daily movement too. As muscle mass and bone density decline, your chances of losing your balance during everyday tasks—from carrying uneven loads (like your workbag) to standing on your toes to reach a high shelf—increase.

What You Can Do:

ADD FLEXIBILITY TRAINING

Flexibility training helps you fix the muscle imbalances caused by everyday life. When one muscle or muscle group is weak or underused, others around it are forced to work harder or in unnatural ways to complete a move, which increases your risk of injury. Flexibility training allows you to address those imbalances with moves that help to reduce strain on overworked muscles and improve your range of motion so you can live—and exercise—with less pain and fewer injuries.

No doubt about it, your body changes as the years go by. It doesn't look or work the way it did in your 20s, but it's not supposed to. Over the decades, your body has let you do many things you loved, perhaps dancing at weddings, playing with your pets, going on adventurous vacations, or hugging your family and friends. Whether your goal is to keep doing what you love or get fitter than ever, one thing is clear: The more you move, the better equipped you will be to handle the challenges that aging throws your way. And that's exactly what this program will help you do. You'll learn how to move efficiently—and safely—so you can age into your strongest years yet.

CHAPTER 2

The Key to Staying Strong as You Age

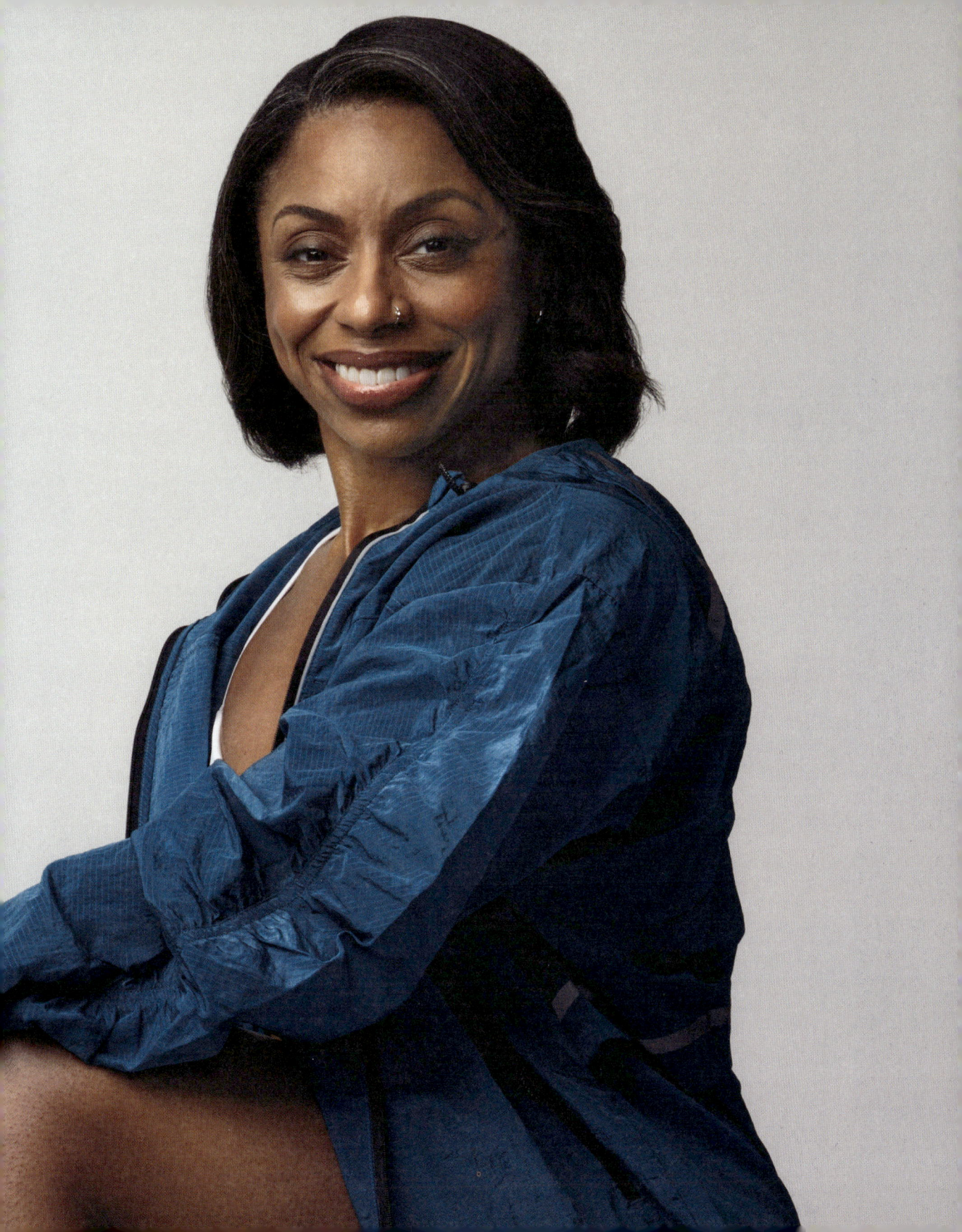

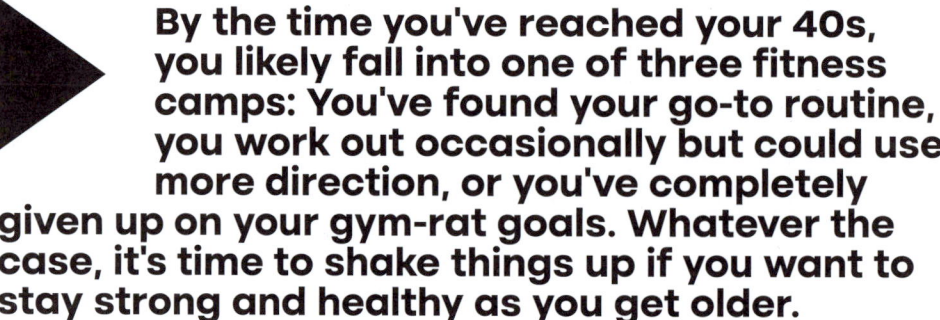 **By the time you've reached your 40s, you likely fall into one of three fitness camps: You've found your go-to routine, you work out occasionally but could use more direction, or you've completely given up on your gym-rat goals. Whatever the case, it's time to shake things up if you want to stay strong and healthy as you get older.**

If you're a regular at the gym, you're already way ahead of the game, but sticking to the same routine can have its pitfalls. Unless your workout includes a wide variety of exercises, there's a chance you're overworking some muscles and underworking others, which can lead to imbalances. Plus, if you easily get bored with your sweat sessions, doing the same routine for years on end can squash motivation. Change it up every now and then so you can ensure you're training all your muscles equally and adding some fun to your fitness. In the 28-day plan, you'll work different muscle groups each day, which keeps workouts enjoyable while minimizing downtime and still giving your muscles ample rest.

If you work out occasionally but struggle to stay consistent, you're well on your path to getting strong and fit. You already know the basics, which means you won't have to spend too much time learning new moves. However, adopting a regular workout schedule is crucial to seeing results. Luckily, this plan will take the guesswork out of what to do each day so you can stay on top of your fitness goals.

Now, if you've fallen off the fitness wagon, don't despair—starting again is easier than you think. Your body has muscle memory, or a physiological blueprint, for all the activities you've ever done (just like riding a bike!). Of course, making the decision to get up and move is just half the battle when you're trying to stay strong. But, what exactly are you supposed to do next?

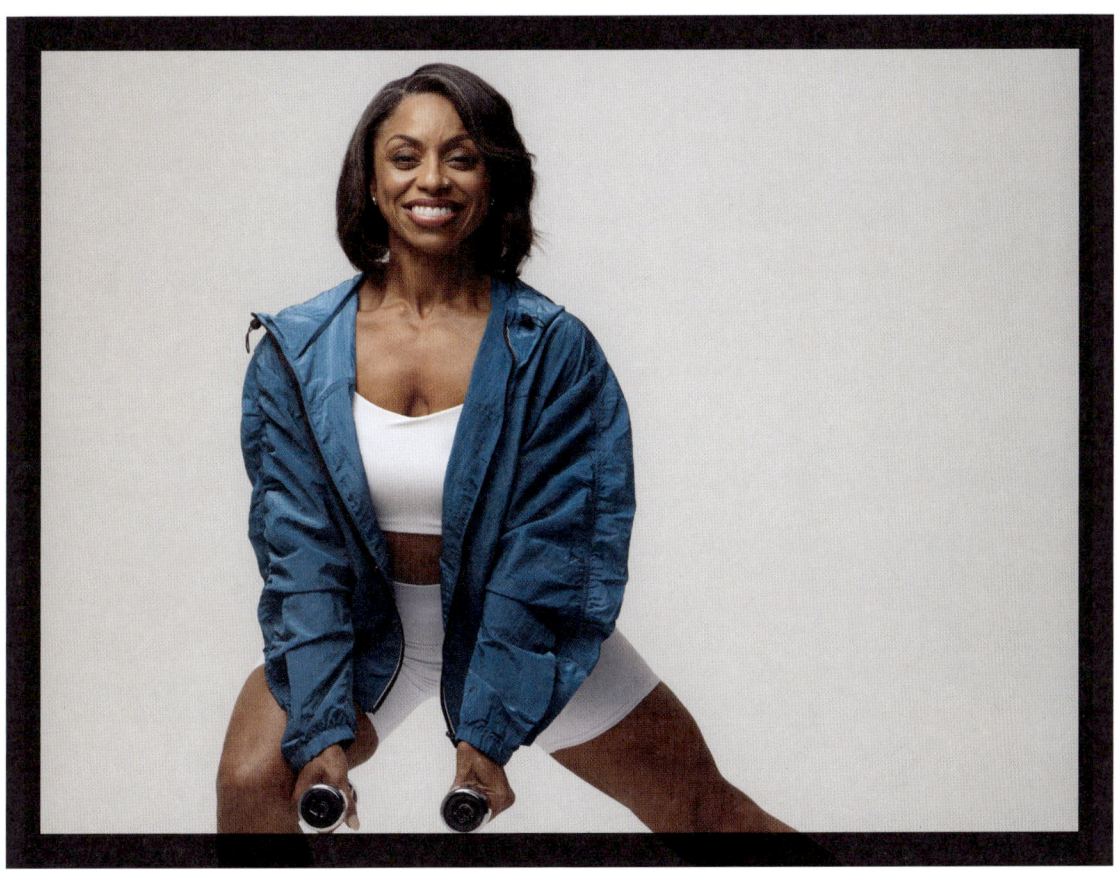

Find the Right Mix of Cardio and Strength

It's one of the top questions trainers are asked time and again: Is cardio or strength training better for overall fitness? As much as we love keeping it simple, the truth is a combination of both are essential for feeling your best in your 40s and beyond.

Cardio is key to improving cardiovascular health, while strength training is nonnegotiable when it comes to maintaining and building muscle. Before we dive into what they have to offer, here's a refresher on what makes each unique.

CARDIO—short for cardiorespiratory training—refers to any exercise that creates such an energy demand on your system that it elevates your heart rate and gets your blood pumping faster, which helps with improving heart and lung health, building endurance, and burning calories. Think: walking, jogging, biking, swimming, and dancing.

STRENGTH TRAINING, on the other hand, involves using your own body weight or tools like dumbbells or resistance bands to build muscle mass and strength. It's proven to be effective at promoting bone density and increasing the overall integrity of connective tissues over time, building lean muscle, and decreasing body fat, leading to a more

The Key to Staying Strong as You Age

CARDIO BEFORE STRENGTH OR VICE VERSA?

If you prefer to do a little bit of both cardio and strength training on the same day, follow this advice recommended by the American Council on Exercise.

- ▶ If your goal is better endurance, do cardio **before** weights.

- ▶ If your goal is burning fat and losing weight, do cardio **after** weights.

- ▶ If you want to get stronger, do cardio **after** weights.

- ▶ On upper-body strength training days, you can do **either first**.

- ▶ On lower-body strength training days, do cardio **after** weights.

- ▶ If your goal is just general fitness, do **either first**, but maybe start with the one you like less.

---

toned and defined physique. Exercises like pushups, biceps curls, and squats all count as strength training.

As you now know, your body changes in all sorts of ways as you age, so to feel your best, you need an exercise routine that supports all parts of your health. Both cardio and strength have their own superpowers, but they really shine when you add a little of both to your routine. Master the right mix—like you'll do in this plan—and here are all the benefits you can expect.

YOU'LL BUILD AND MAINTAIN MUSCLE MASS

Lifting increasingly larger amounts of weight signals your muscles to adapt and grow bigger and/or stronger making strength training the ideal defense against muscle loss. It'll also help target muscles you don't normally use when you're doing cardio.

But you can't strength train every day and expect to get stronger. Your muscles need time off to repair themselves—that's how they grow. However, that doesn't mean you have to put your fitness goals on pause. Mixing cardio into your weekly workout schedule gives your muscles a break from resistance training without messing with your momentum. (You should still take at least one true rest day per week, but more on that later.) Plus, the boost to your heart and lungs you'll get can help make pumping out higher rep counts a little easier as your endurance improves.

YOU'LL IMPROVE YOUR BODY COMPOSITION

Cardio might be the first thing to come to mind when you think of exercising for weight loss. But you'll get more fat-burning benefits when you combine cardio training with strength training. Doing so creates an opportunity for your body to burn calories at an elevated rate even after you're done exercising as your body works to recover and repair its muscles. This fitness phenomenon is formally known as excess postexercise oxygen consumption (EPOC).

The muscle you'll gain from strength training also requires more calories to maintain than fat, giving you an added burn even at rest. So the more muscles you maintain—and build—the more energy it requires, so you'll burn more fat all day long. When you build more muscle and decrease body fat, you'll see a more defined and toned physique overall.

YOU'LL INCREASE ENERGY AND ENDURANCE

Whatever ways you want to be able to move your body in the years to come, cardio and strength training can help power it. Want to chase your kids or nieces and nephews without getting winded? Cardio helps your body more efficiently transport oxygen to your muscles and build strong lungs. In turn, you'll be able to

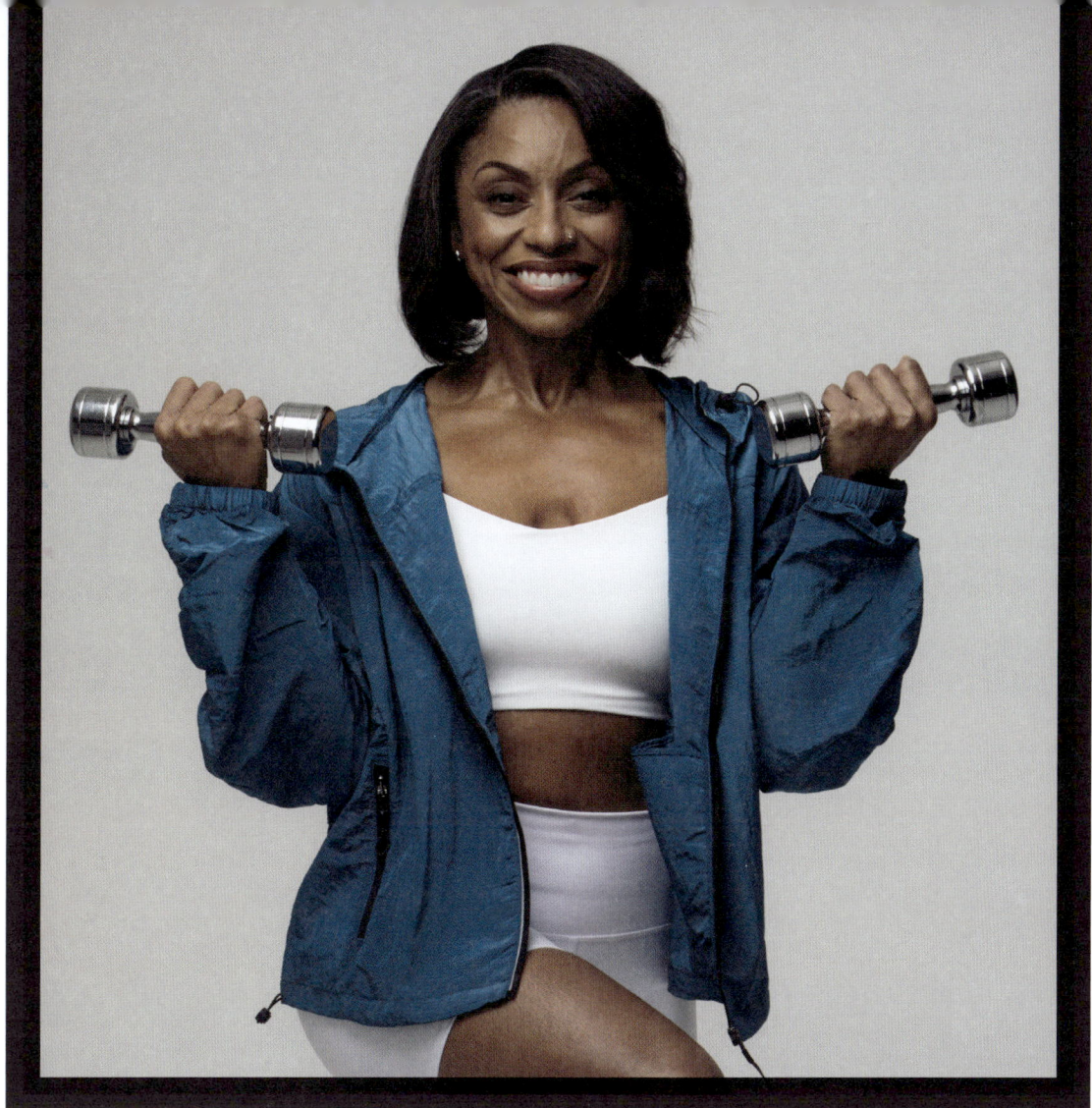

run around for longer without needing a break, thanks to a steady supply of oxygen. Want to hike, travel, and explore? The muscle you'll build strength training will keep you feeling strong as you climb stairs, trek up hills, and haul luggage. Better yet, cardio can actually increase your energy supply due to the creation of mitochondria. Consider it a one-two punch for feeling your best all day, every day.

YOU'LL STRENGTHEN YOUR JOINTS

Any weight-bearing workout will actually help strengthen the muscles surrounding your joints to stabilize them. As a personal trainer who lives with rheumatoid arthritis, Coach Ash recommends doing exercises using weights (dumbbells, kettlebells, resistance bands, etc.), like farmer's carries or shoulder presses, that mimic functional movement patterns such as carrying groceries or reaching for something from the top shelf of your cabinet. By doing these exercises, you'll help keep your core, arms, and shoulders healthy while also training your body to handle everyday activities with ease. And pairing it with a cardio workout like swimming, where you have to overcome the resistance of the water, can boost joint-strengthening results while reducing your risk of injury.

It's clear the right combo of cardio and strength training can amp up your overall fitness, but exactly how much of each should you do? It depends on your individual goals, but in this plan we recommend focusing more on strength and supplementing it with a day of low-impact cardio as active recovery. At the end of the day, it's more important that you do what gets you excited and makes you feel good. Just make sure to tune in to how your body responds to the movements you do so you can adjust as needed and keep going strong.

Work Hard, Rest Hard

Can't commit to a daily workout? That's actually not a problem! Staying fit doesn't require as much time as you think. Striking a balance between challenging training sessions and time for recovery may seem tricky, but fitness pros have some clear advice about how often you should work out—and what types of exercise you should focus on when you do.

The U.S. Department of Health recommends at least 150 minutes (2 hours and 30 minutes) of moderate physical activity a week, but you typically only need to work out a minimum of three days per week to see results, up to six days max, regardless of your goal.

As for what you can do on those three to six days? It's all about striking a balance between cardio and strength. Remember: Cardio is any activity that gets your heart rate up and blood pumping faster. And adding some strength training to your routine could be as simple as grabbing some water bottles and trying a few biceps curls, arm circles, or lateral extensions, says De Bolton, a NASM-certified personal trainer, corrective exercise specialist, and weight-loss specialist, of FaithFueled Moms.

Taking it a step further, Coach Ash built the 28 days of her program to focus on different muscle groups each day, breaking it up between upper body, lower body, core, and full body, while adding cardio and active but low-impact recovery days. This routine checks every box: It has strength training to build muscle, cardio to maintain your endurance and cardiovascular health, and core exercises to help with balance and mobility.

Coach Ash also built in a day for true rest. Taking the time completely off from your workouts is just as important to getting fit as giving your all to every rep and set. Soon after beginning this program, you'll start seeing results and may feel motivated to do more. Just remember that your muscles also need time to recover and adapt so you continue to grow stronger as you age.

Once we get into the program, you'll notice that the number of days you work out per week gradually increases. We'll start slow, then build up each week as your body gets stronger and can handle more. However, by working different muscle groups each day, we'll make sure you're not overtraining. For example: In Week 1, you'll torch your upper body on Tuesday, do some active recovery on Wednesday, then work your lower body on Thursday, giving your upper body plenty of time to recharge. This way, you maximize your efforts on the mat and progress faster without the fatigue that usually comes with a daily workout.

Bounce Back Stronger

Taking a break from working out each week is just one piece of the puzzle when it comes to restoring your energy. There are also plenty of ways to boost the benefits of your time off so you return to your routine feeling unstoppable. And that's especially important after age 40, when workout recovery can take a bit longer than in decades past. With muscle mass, bone density,

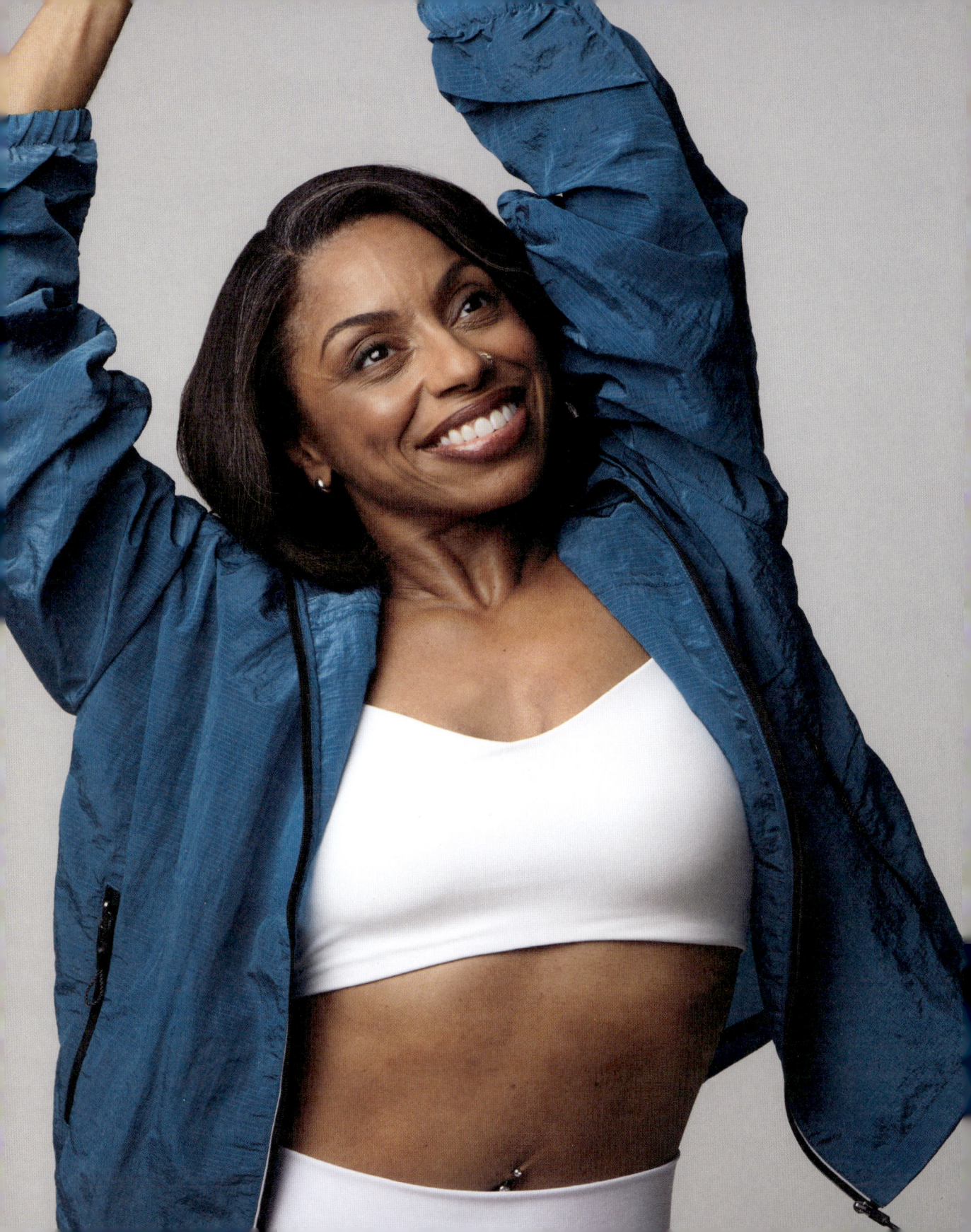

YOUR FEEL-GOOD STRETCHING ROUTINE

As we age, it's important to get a stretch in after each workout to head off soreness and recover faster. Not sure how to go about it? Here's Coach Ash's favorite stretching combo:

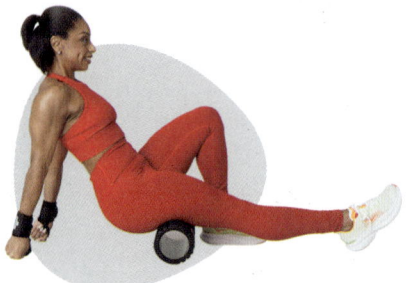

FOAM ROLLING

▶ Start with foam rolling. Use gentle pressure and slow, controlled movements to roll out each muscle group for 1 to 2 minutes, focusing on any tight or sore areas.

▶ Then, run through the following moves, holding each for 20 to 30 seconds:

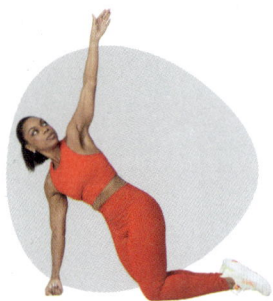

T-SPINE ROTATION (P.124)

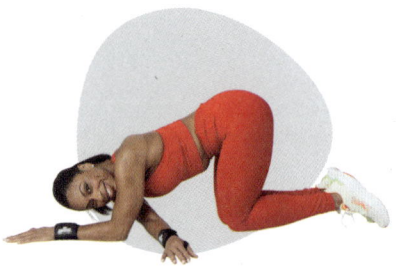

THREAD THE NEEDLE (P.125)

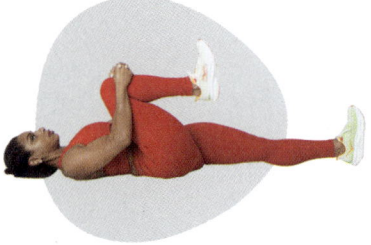

LYING HIP FLEXOR STRETCH (P.110)

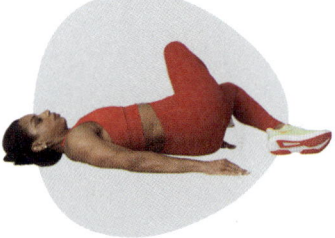

FIGURE FOUR TO TWIST (P.104)

and estrogen levels all on the decline, you might need more than a good night's rest to feel replenished.

If you want to see the best results possible from your workouts—and protect your body from future harm, you'll need to make time to recover properly. The good news is that the most tried-and-true tactics are easy to do and fit into your everyday routines.

Here's how you can amp up your recovery and power through every workout with ease.

After Every Single Workout

Do at least 10 minutes of these two classics.

STRETCHING

Stretching is essential for maintaining flexibility, preventing injuries, and ensuring your muscles recover properly. It's not just about reaching further—it's about giving your body the care it needs to perform at its best every day, says Coach Ash. In addition to lengthening your muscles (which tighten during exercise), stretching boosts circulation, helping to deliver oxygen and other nutrients needed for healing from exercise, says Austin Martinez, ATC, director of education for Stretch Lab Franchise, a studio that specializes in flexibility training. Oh, and it's free. For the ultimate feel-good stretch after every workout, try Coach Ash's go-to routine on page 24.

FOAM ROLLING

Much like massage, foam rolling (a.k.a. self-myofascial release, or SMR) signals your nervous system to chill. "It's the simplest, most cost-effective way to decrease muscle tension and related joint pain," says Rick Richey, DHSc, cofounder of Rēcover, a studio in New York City that's dedicated to fitness prehab and rehab. It also improves your range of motion and minimizes soreness, according to research. To massage a muscle, position it on top of your roller and move back and forth lengthwise a few times, Richey says. As you roll, feel for tender spots. Roll out each muscle group for 1 to 2 minutes.

When Your Body Needs a Little Extra TLC

After the basics, layer in additional tools if you're sorer than usual or when you start to really intensify your workouts.

PERCUSSIVE THERAPY

Curious about those massage guns that everyone on your feed is pounding their muscles with? They're totally legit. If foam rolling is not your jam for your recovery needs, percussive therapy is a fantastic alternative. Massage guns can help relieve muscle soreness, improve circulation, and enhance flexibility, providing a deeper, more targeted massage that promotes faster recovery and better performance. Coach Ash personally prefers this method to relieve rheumatoid arthritis aches and pains.

BATHS

An oldie but a super goodie, Epsom salt (a.k.a. magnesium) soaks will ramp up your recovery efforts. The calming effect of an aromatic bath can definitely help your body relax and enter a recovery state to alleviate muscle aches, says Coach Ash. Plus, studies also show that a hot bath or shower before bed improves sleep, which is crucial for recovery. Soak for 10 to 20 minutes whenever your mind and body need a break.

When You're Really Exhausted

Crush a workout, conquer the world—right? A good sweat makes us feel all the things: unstoppable, sexy, strong. But, as with Netflix dramas and fiber-filled veggies, too much of a good thing applies to your fitness routine as well.

The workout schedule in this plan is designed to gradually build your strength by starting you off slowly and easily, focusing on the basics and getting your body used to proper form so you can head off injuries as you progressively add load. Soon, you'll feel the satisfaction of these workouts and you may feel like wanting to push more and more. And that's partly what this program aims to do:

get you so excited about working out and feeling your strongest self yet.

But here's the inconvenient truth about wanting to do more: Though we tend to associate it solely with feel-good endorphins, exercise—especially high-intensity or endurance training—triggers a stress response in our bodies, spiking fight-or-flight hormones like cortisol, says Stacy Sims, PhD, a *WH* advisor and the author of *Roar: How to Match Your Food and Fitness to Your Female Physiology for Optimum Performance, Great Health, and a Strong, Lean Body for Life*. This reaction is okay (in fact, it's what signals your body to ultimately get stronger or faster)—unless you don't have time to recover from it. Throw in a little cortisol-elevating life stress on top of those nonstop all-out workouts, and you can expect your fitness to pay the price.

Listen to your body so you know when you're starting to feel a little more run down than usual and try the following tips to help you keep moving for longer.

CHOOSE STRENGTH OVER INTENSITY

Ease up on any of your HIIT, hardcore cardio, and CrossFit-style workouts, all of which demand cortisol, according to trainer and nutritional therapy practitioner Emily Schromm, CPT. "You have to give yourself permission to take it from 100 percent to 60 percent," she says. That way, you can transition from a state of breakdown to one of repair. Instead, set your sights on strength, since it has a minimal effect on cortisol levels. Opt for a weight with which you can only perform 4 to 6 reps per set.

FIND AN ANCHOR

Remember your *why*. Get outside, sans smart watch. Reconnect to doing certain activities without the pressure of hitting a specific time goal or reps count. Shift the focus off your stats and have fun.

DISCOVER NEW WAYS TO CHILL OUT

If sweating is your sole outlet after a rough day, explore other options for finding peace. Though they can still involve being in motion, they don't have to be strenuous workouts, says Coach Ash. Some of her favorite ways to recharge include leisurely walks outdoors, relaxing in the pool, stretching, meditating, deep breathing, and journaling.

Stay Hyped Your Whole Workout

Rallying the motivation to work out can be a huge hurdle at times. On the days when you're dragging, try these tips to stay happy and inspired from your warm-up to your final rep.

TREAT YOURSELF TO A LITTLE R&R FIRST

▶ Here's your plan: Relax with your number one episode of *Friends* and then go sweat. Yes, really.

If you're feeling totally depleted, watching a rerun of your favorite show may actually boost your willpower to get things done, according to research by the University of Buffalo. (This isn't permission for a Netflix binge, though; cue up one episode then go work out. Just one.)

50%

That's how much you can reduce muscle soreness by foam rolling after a workout.

Source: *Frontiers in Physiology*

LISTEN TO THAT PODCAST EVERYONE'S TALKING ABOUT

▶ Make workout time more enticing by pairing it with something you actually want to do—like finally catching up on that podcast your coworker keeps raving about.

This strategy is called temptation bundling. Katherine Milkman, PhD, an associate professor at The Wharton School at the University of Pennsylvania, dreamed it up. After studying students who wanted to work out more, she found that those who could only access audiobooks at the gym were 29 percent more likely to work out than those who could access audiobooks whenever. They were also 51 percent more likely to exercise than students who were given $25 and told to work out more.

GIVE YOURSELF THE RIGHT KIND OF PEP TALK

▶ Self-talk is often hyped as a motivational tool, but you've got to do it right to really reap the benefits. Research suggests that talking to yourself in the second person is actually more effective than chatting yourself up in the first.

So next time you're feeling sluggish, tell yourself, "You're going to crush this next set," instead of "I will crush this next set," or "You got this, woman," instead of "I can do this."

REPLAY YOUR PERSONAL FITNESS HIGHLIGHTS REEL

▶ Remember that time you absolutely crushed that boot camp workout and felt like a superhero afterward? Envision that memory the next time you're staring down the dumbbells.

In one University of New Hampshire study, participants asked to think about positive exercise memories had higher levels of subsequent exercise than those who didn't take a trip down memory lane. In other words, the more you can associate positive emotions with working out, the more likely you are to show up.

CUE UP THE RIGHT PLAYLIST

▶ Whether you need a good pump-up song to get you started or jam to motivate you through the last stretch of your workout, high-energy music can take you from couch to crushing it in three minutes flat.

Max out your playlist by choosing songs that have 125 to 140 beats per minute. (That's about as fast as Britney Spears's "Work B**ch.") Research published in *Science of Sport and Exercise* suggests it's the optimal tempo for keeping your head in the game and feeling motivated.

ENLIST YOURSELF A SUPER-FIT WORKOUT BUDDY

▶ Working out with someone you perceive as more physically fit than you can help you increase your workout time and intensity by 200 percent, according to research out of Kansas State University. So grab that workout buddy ASAP.

With the right workout, recovery, and motivation, it's totally possible to get and stay fit as you add more candles to your birthday cake every year. Plus, when you follow a plan that does the heavy lifting by building in those game-changing details (the best strength exercises, the perfect mix of rest days, and everything else), feeling next-level fit in your 40s and beyond is really a no-brainer. All that's left to do is get started!

CHAPTER 3

The 28-Day Plan

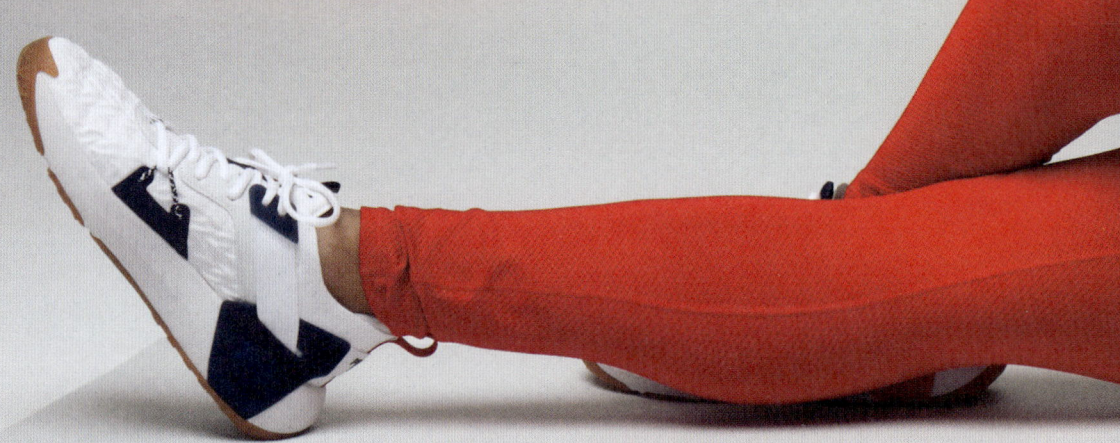

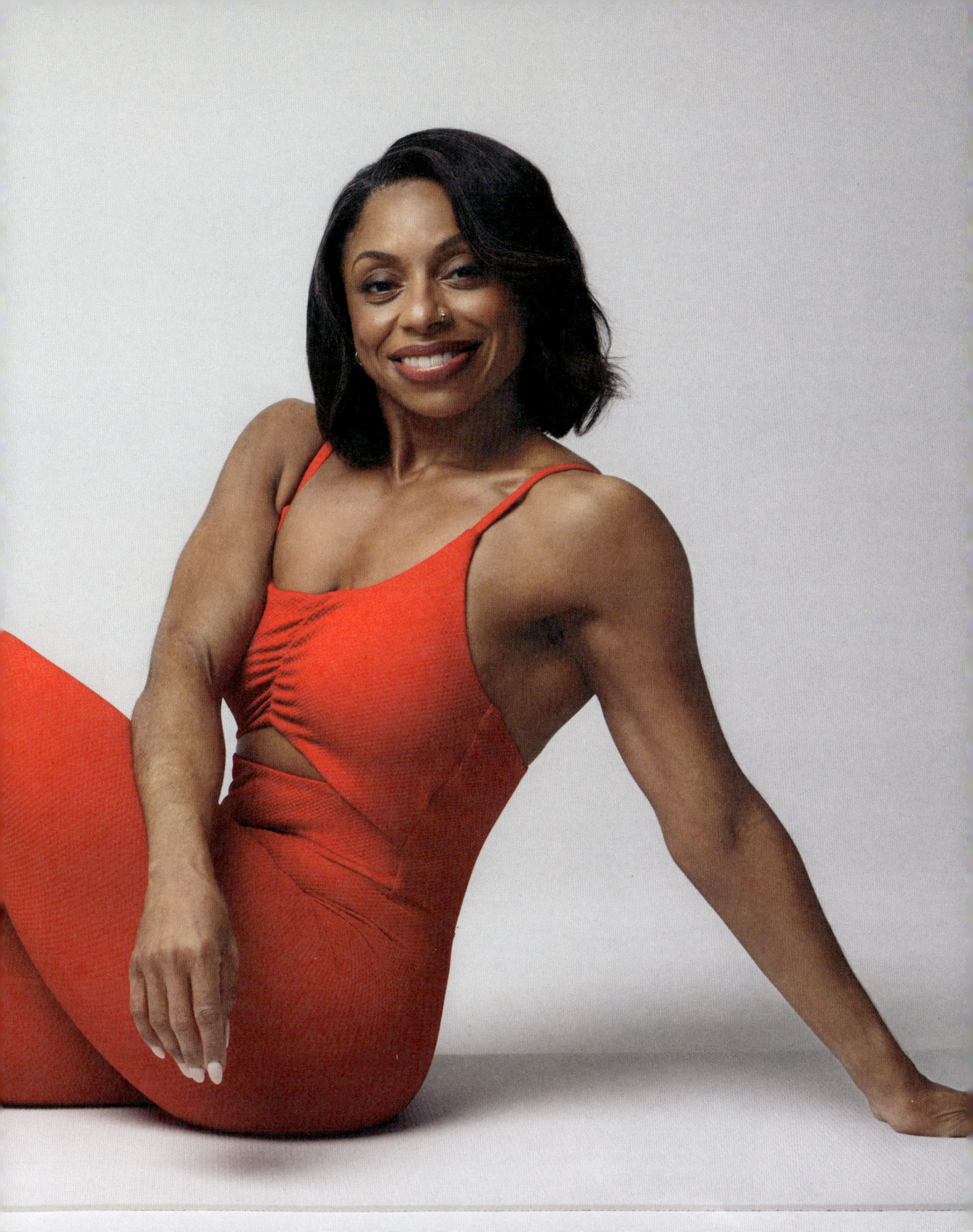

Welcome To Your 28-Day Strength-Training Plan!

▶ This program is designed specifically to address the unique challenges that women over 40 face such as hormonal changes, slower metabolism, and joint pain. Each day of the plan has a specific theme, focusing on different muscle groups to ensure a balanced approach to fitness. With four or five days dedicated to strength training and two or three days for active recovery or rest, this plan aims to build muscle, enhance joint stability, and improve overall fitness in a manageable and effective way.

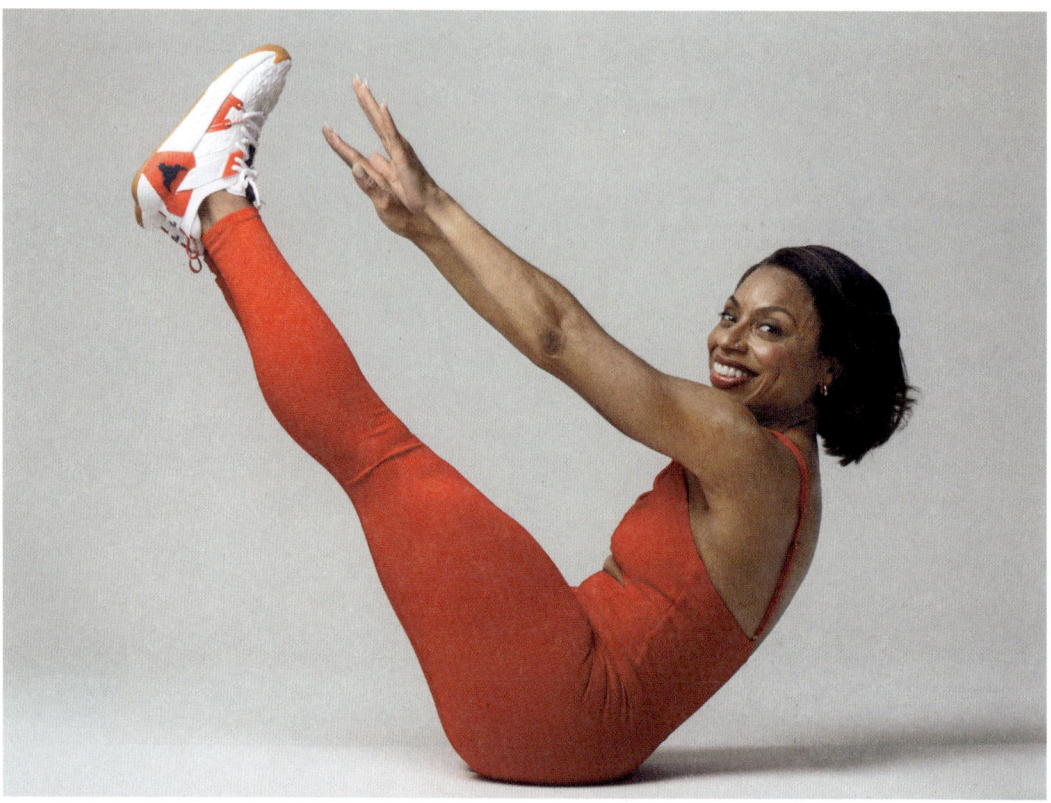

What You Can Expect Each Week

Each day's workout focuses on a different muscle group to ensure a comprehensive strength-training regimen. You'll start the program working out four days each week. The rest of the week, you have the option to truly rest or engage in some light cardio for active recovery. In Week 2, we encourage you to increase active recovery to two days and have one true rest day.

At this point, you'll start to feel you're able to handle a little bit more, so workout days will increase to five days, and you'll have one true rest day and one day for active recovery.

This is what your week could look like:

MONDAY Full-Body Strength

TUESDAY Upper-Body Strength

WEDNESDAY Rest or Active Recovery

THURSDAY Lower-Body Strength

FRIDAY Core and Stability

SATURDAY Rest and Rejuvenate

SUNDAY Rest or Light Cardio

Progressive Workouts

The workouts will change slightly each week, either by adding another set or increasing the weights used, ensuring continuous improvement. Each session can be completed in 30 minutes or less, making it easy to fit into a busy schedule. Prioritizing dynamic stretching before the workout helps to prepare your muscles and joints, reducing the risk of injury. Examples of dynamic stretches include leg swings, arm circles, and torso twists. Coach Ash has built in an efficient routine to get you primed for your daily workouts in the 28-day plan, but feel free to add some of these dynamic stretches for an extended warm-up if you need it. After your workout, focus on static stretching to aid in recovery and flexibility, such as holding a hamstring stretch or a quad stretch for 30 seconds. Or try Coach Ash's Feel-Good Stretching Routine on page 24 to take the guesswork out of recovering faster.

Active Recovery and the Importance of Rest

Active recovery is crucial for muscle repair and growth. On active recovery days, engage in light activities that promote blood flow without straining your muscles. Examples include a brisk 15-minute walk, light cycling, or gentle yoga poses like child's pose and cat-cow stretch. These activities help reduce muscle soreness and improve flexibility. Rest days are equally important. They allow your muscles to recover and grow stronger. Overtraining can lead to fatigue, decreased performance, and even injury. Ensure you listen to your body and take full advantage of rest days to rejuvenate both physically and mentally.

After 28 Days

It's essential to maintain the momentum upon completing this program. One effective way is to cycle through the program again, continuing to increase weights or sets as you progress. Alternatively, you can integrate new exercises or join a fitness class to keep things fresh and challenging. The key is consistency and variety to prevent plateaus and keep your muscles engaged. Remember, movement is medicine! Motion is lotion! Keep moving!

WHAT YOU'LL NEED

One of the great aspects of this program is that all workouts can be done at home with minimal equipment.

- A yoga mat
- A set of dumbbells (light, medium, and heavy)
- Resistance band loops (light, medium, and heavy)
- A water bottle and towel
- A pair of medium-weight kettlebells (optional)

Light dumbbells should range from 2 to 5 pounds, medium dumbbells from 8 to 12 pounds, and heavy dumbbells from 15 pounds and up.

While you can take this program to the gym if you want, it's specifically built to be done at home with very little gear. By following this plan, you'll develop sustainable fitness habits, enhance your strength, and improve your overall health and mobility.

Supercharge Your Workouts

As you begin working your way through this plan, you'll start slow and focus on proper form. Help your body along with these tips to boost your results and feel energized through every single rep.

GET MOVING
It's easy to feel like you've earned a day on the sofa scrolling through your phone after a sweat session. But if you're able to muster a bit of energy, get up and move instead. Light activity is a great recovery tool because it keeps blood moving, helping you bounce back by repairing and refueling your body.

Plan some light activity throughout the day, even if you are headed to work. Get up, walk around, do some gentle stretches while standing, and breathe deeply. Moving not only helps you recover more quickly, but it also keeps your body primed for the next workout.

PRIORITIZE SLEEP
Muscle growth takes place during recovery periods. And much of that recovery takes place during sleep. Exercisers who receive fewer than six hours of sleep per night have less strength than those who get seven or more hours of sleep nightly, according to a Chinese study from the *Journal of Musculoskeletal and Neuronal Interactions*.

Suffering from insomnia or sleep interruptions related to hormone changes and menopause? Head that off by setting up a healthy sleep environment which may involve relaxing activities before bed, reducing screen time, investing in blackout curtains (or an eye mask to keep the faintest of light out), and keeping the thermostat at an optimally cool temperature (between 65 and 67 degrees).

PACK ON PROTEIN
Humans need amino acids, the building blocks of protein, to make sure every structure of the body— bone, liver, gut, tissues, hair, nails, skin, and muscles—functions optimally. And there are benefits to consuming protein—a non-negotiable for building muscle—before and after workouts.

Protein primes your muscles to put in the work. So if you're prepping for an extra tough workout (which you might encounter halfway through the plan), research suggests that protein supports muscle endurance to keep you feeling strong. Meanwhile, consuming protein within two hours of working out can aid in the process of muscle repair and growth. Aim for 20 to 30 grams of protein at every meal, and you'll set yourself up for muscle-building success.

HYDRATE, HYDRATE, HYDRATE
Going into a workout even mildly dehydrated can negatively impact exercise performance. The American Council on Exercise recommends drinking 17 to 20 ounces of water two to three hours before exercise, and another eight ounces of water 20 to 30 minutes after the workout.

Hydrating *during* your workouts is important, too, since you lose fluids through sweating. If you don't feel that thirsty, drink anyway. Drinking smaller amounts at regular intervals can help you absorb fluid more effectively and avoid stomach sloshing.

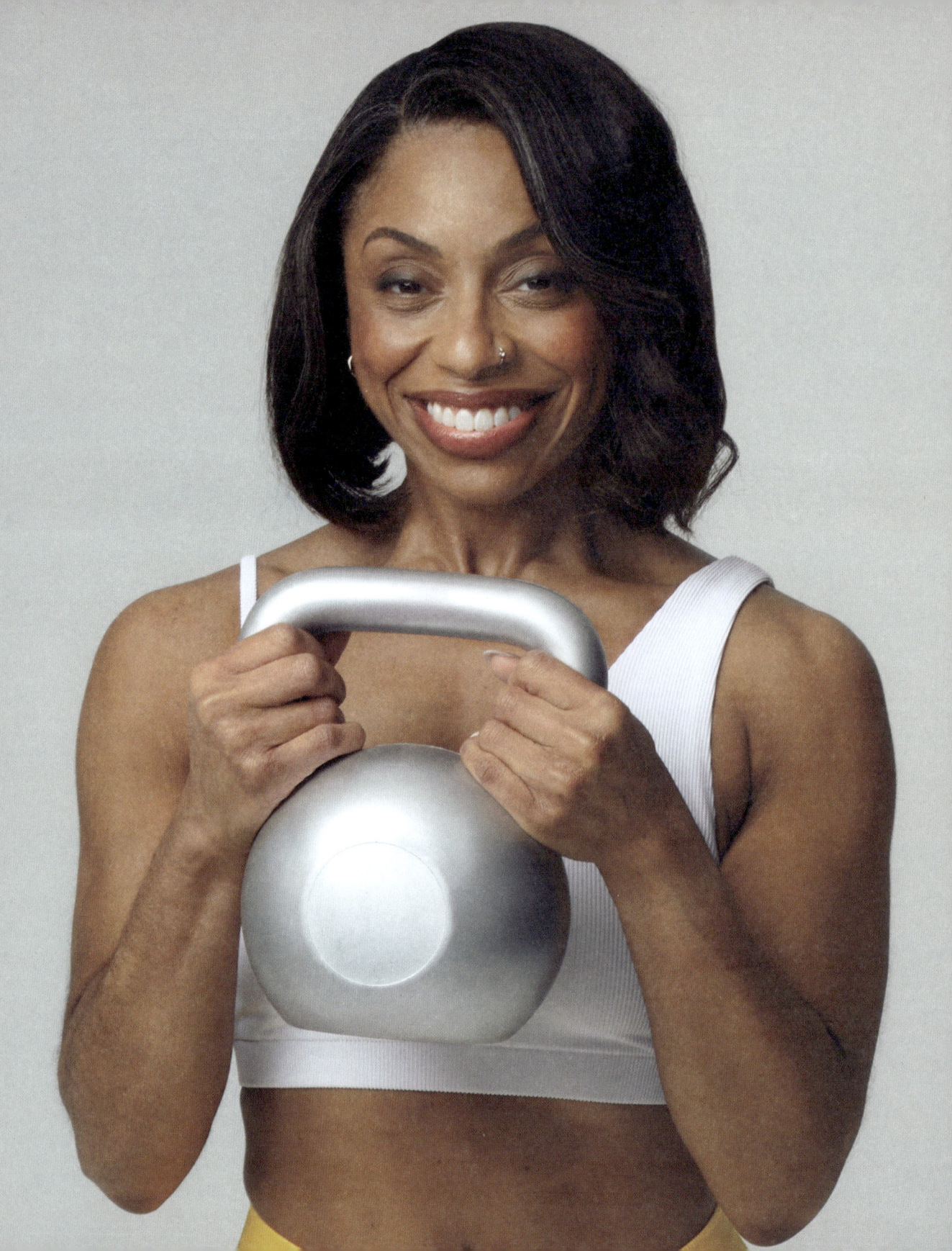

WEEK 1 At A Glance

▶ **DAY 1** Full-Body Strength

▶ **DAY 2** Upper-Body Strength

▶ **DAY 3** Rest or Active Recovery

▶ **DAY 4** Lower-Body Strength

▶ **DAY 5** Core and Stability

▶ **DAY 6** Rest and Rejuvenate

▶ **DAY 7** Rest or Light Cardio

TRACK YOUR PROGRESS

As you go through your plan each week, the thumbnails are there to make it easy for you to follow along with the exercises. If you need more guidance, turn to the exercise guide (page number noted for each) to learn exactly how to do these moves. Remember to jot down any training notes as well as what weight you used for each move and each set in the space provided so you can make adjustments along the way and feel good about the progress you're making.

WEEK 1 Day 1
Full-Body Strength

WARM-UP

Perform each exercise for 30 seconds, resting 10 seconds between moves. After completing all moves, rest for one minute then repeat the circuit.

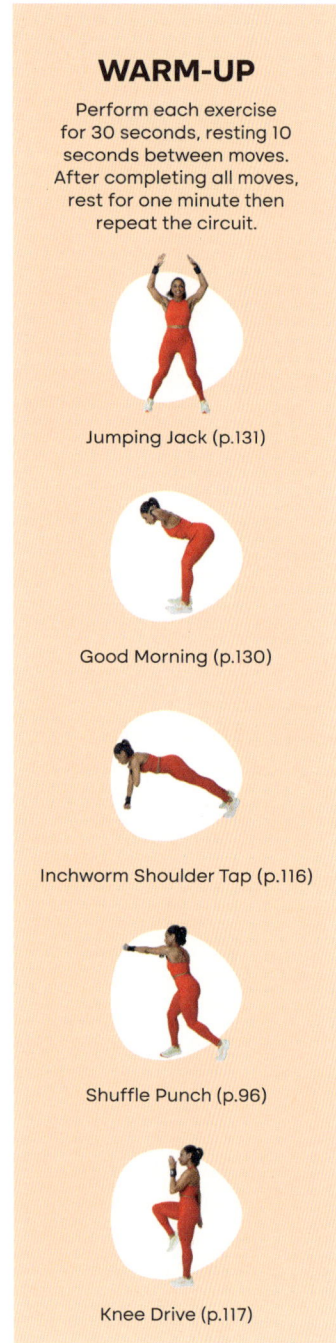

Jumping Jack (p.131)

Good Morning (p.130)

Inchworm Shoulder Tap (p.116)

Shuffle Punch (p.96)

Knee Drive (p.117)

EXERCISE

Exercise	
SQUAT TO OVERHEAD PRESS (P.138) ▶ Light to medium dumbbells	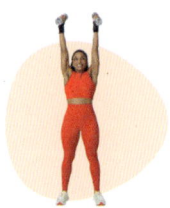
DEADLIFT AND ROW (P.136) ▶ Medium dumbbells	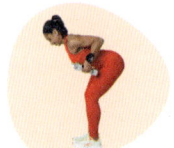
CURTSY LUNGE WITH BICEPS CURL (P.134) ▶ Light to medium dumbbells	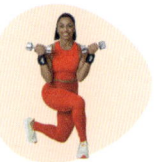
SIDE LUNGE AND ROW (P.135) ▶ Medium dumbbells	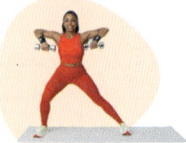
SQUAT AND SNATCH (P.137) ▶ Medium dumbbell	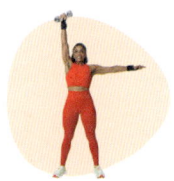
DEADBUG (P.113) ▶ Body weight	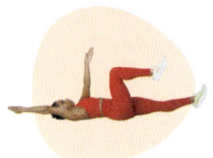

▶ **REST** Rest 20 seconds between each exercise and 45 seconds between sets.

WORK	SET 1	SET 2	SET 3
10 reps			
10 reps			
10 reps per side			
10 reps per side			
10 reps per side			
10 reps per side, alternating			

WEEK 1 Day 2
Upper-Body Strength

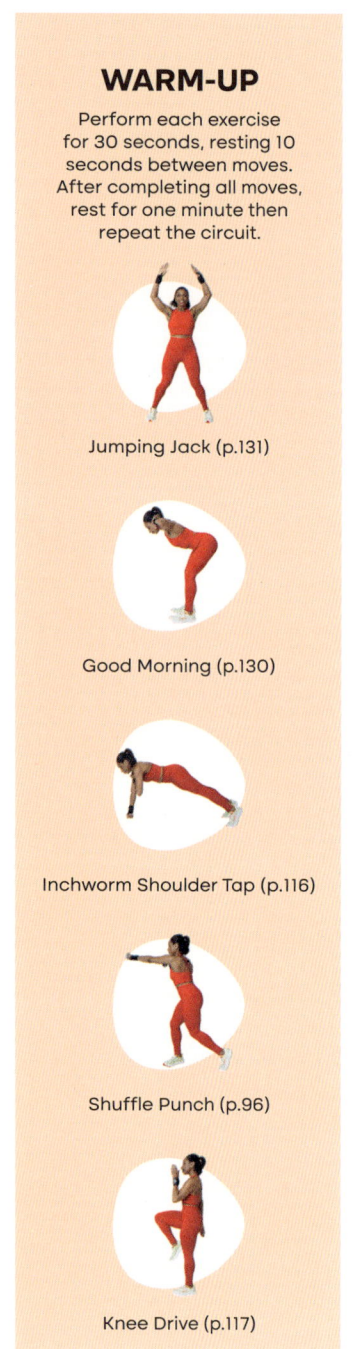

WARM-UP

Perform each exercise for 30 seconds, resting 10 seconds between moves. After completing all moves, rest for one minute then repeat the circuit.

- Jumping Jack (p.131)
- Good Morning (p.130)
- Inchworm Shoulder Tap (p.116)
- Shuffle Punch (p.96)
- Knee Drive (p.117)

EXERCISE

Exercise	
WARRIOR ONE ROW (P.127) ▶ Medium dumbbells	
SINGLE SINGLE DOUBLE BICEPS CURL (P.91) ▶ Light dumbbells	
ISOMETRIC LATERAL RAISE (P.99) ▶ Light dumbbells	
BRIDGE CHEST PRESS (P.95) ▶ Medium dumbbells	
TRICEPS KICKBACK (P.94) ▶ Light dumbbells	
REAR DELT FLY (P.93) ▶ Light dumbbells	

▶ **REST** Rest 20 seconds between each exercise and 45 seconds between sets.

WORK	SET 1	SET 2	SET 3
10 reps per side			
10 reps			
Hold first rep 5 sec., then 10 reps more holding 5-10 sec.			
10 reps			
10 reps			
10 reps			

The 28-Day Plan

WEEK 1 Day 3
Rest or Active Recovery

YOUR CHOICE
Use this day to rest your body or do this active recovery routine.

EXERCISE

GOOD MORNING (P.130)
▶ Body weight

90/90 TAP (P.112)
▶ Body weight

DEADBUG (P.113)
▶ Body weight

CHILD'S POSE (P.129)
▶ Body weight

LIGHT CARDIO OF CHOICE (I.E., WALKING, CYCLING, ETC.)

▶ **REST** Rest 30 seconds between each exercise.

WORK	SET 1
15 reps	
15 reps	
15 reps per side, alternating	
30 sec.	
10–15 min.	

WALK YOUR WAY HEALTHY

Walking is a low-impact cardio activity that can make a big impact on your health. Take a stroll and you can:

IMPROVE YOUR MOOD
"Walking and taking deep breaths is a great way to slow your nervous system and get into a relaxed state," says Bradee Felton, CPT, a holistic health coach.

SUPPORT YOUR HEART
Walking at least 40 minutes two or three times a week at an average or brisk pace was associated with a reduced risk of developing heart failure in postmenopausal women, as per a 2018 observational study in the *Journal of the American College of Cardiology*.

INCREASE LONGEVITY
According to the American Heart Association, there's new research that suggests adding just 1,000 steps to your daily routine could lead to a longer life. Not only does it promote heart health, but it also reduces your risk of chronic diseases like obesity, hypertension, and diabetes if you're prediabetic.

WEEK 1 Day 4
Lower-Body Strength

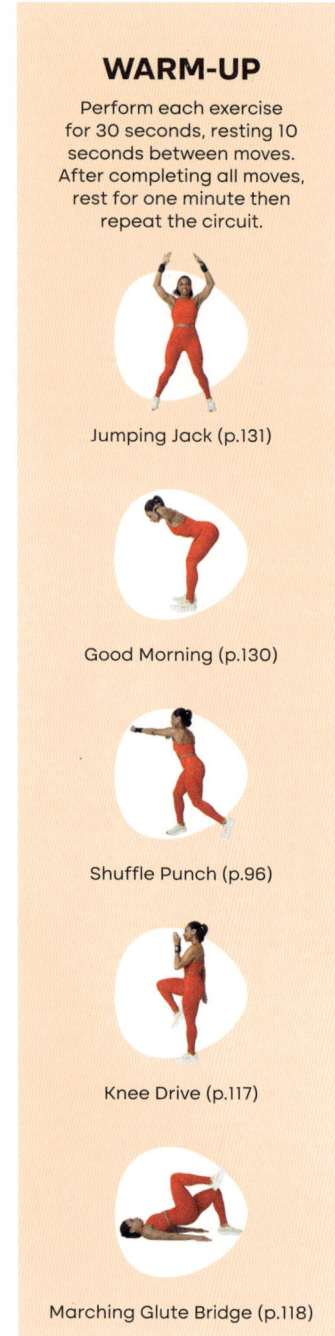

WARM-UP

Perform each exercise for 30 seconds, resting 10 seconds between moves. After completing all moves, rest for one minute then repeat the circuit.

- Jumping Jack (p.131)
- Good Morning (p.130)
- Shuffle Punch (p.96)
- Knee Drive (p.117)
- Marching Glute Bridge (p.118)

EXERCISE

REVERSE LUNGE (P.105)
▶ Medium to heavy dumbbells

DUMBBELL SUMO SQUAT (P.108)
▶ Heavy dumbbell

STAGGERED-STANCE DEADLIFT (P.103)
▶ Medium to heavy dumbbells

BANDED GLUTE BRIDGE (P.101)
▶ Medium to heavy resistance band

CLAMSHELL (P.102)
▶ Medium to heavy resistance band

FOOTBALL SHUFFLE (P.106)
▶ Light to medium resistance band

▶ **REST** Rest 20 seconds between each exercise and 45 seconds between sets.

WORK	SET 1	SET 2	SET 3
10 reps per side			
10 reps			
10 reps per side			
12 reps			
12 reps per side			
20 sec.			

WEEK 1 Day 5
Core and Stability

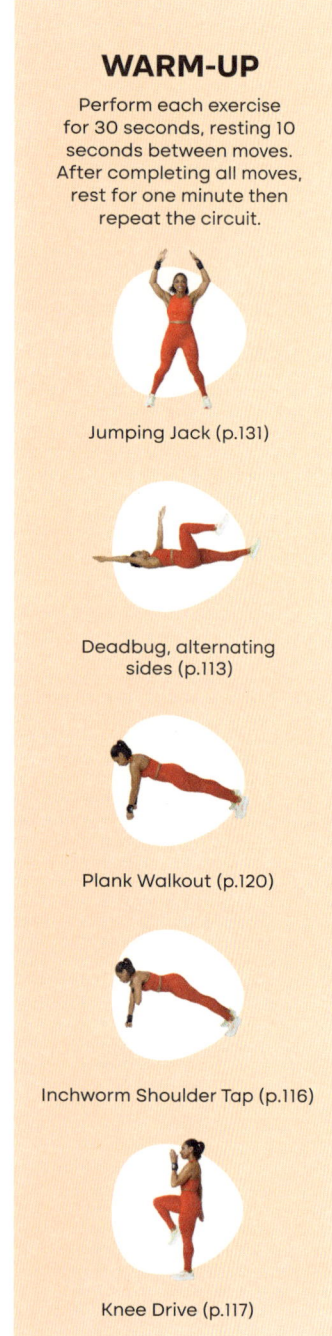

WARM-UP

Perform each exercise for 30 seconds, resting 10 seconds between moves. After completing all moves, rest for one minute then repeat the circuit.

- Jumping Jack (p.131)
- Deadbug, alternating sides (p.113)
- Plank Walkout (p.120)
- Inchworm Shoulder Tap (p.116)
- Knee Drive (p.117)

EXERCISE

V-UP (P.126)
▶ Body weight

MOUNTAIN CLIMBER (P.119)
▶ Body weight

SCISSOR KICK (P.122)
▶ Body weight

SUPERMAN (P.123)
▶ Body weight

FARMER'S CARRY (P.115)
▶ Medium to heavy dumbbells or kettlebells

MODIFIED BURPEE (P.132)
▶ Light dumbbells

▶ **REST** Rest 20 seconds between each exercise and 45 seconds between sets.

WORK	SET 1	SET 2
12 reps		
12 reps		
12 reps		
12 reps		
20 steps		
10 reps		

Day 6
Rest and Rejuvenate

▶ Take today completely off from working out— you deserve it!

Day 7
Rest or Light Cardio

▶ Take today off or do some light cardio, such as walking for 20 minutes, light cycling for 10 to 15 minutes, or stretching for as long as it feels good.

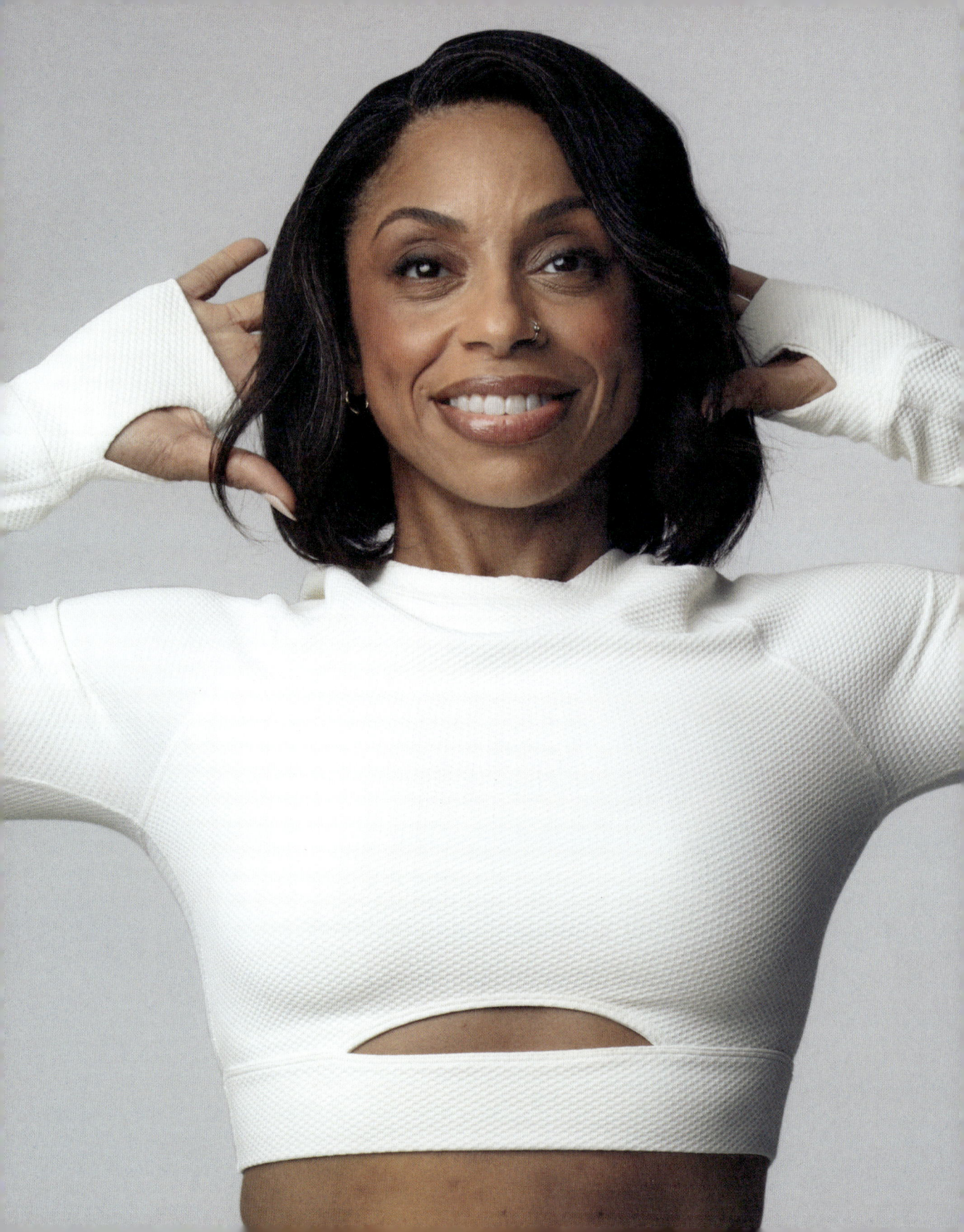

WEEK 2 At A Glance

▶ **DAY 8** Full-Body Strength

▶ **DAY 9** Upper-Body Strength

▶ **DAY 10** Rest or Active Recovery

▶ **DAY 11** Lower-Body Strength

▶ **DAY 12** Rest or Active Recovery

▶ **DAY 13** Full-Body Circuit

▶ **DAY 14** Rest or Light Cardio

TRACK YOUR PROGRESS

As you go through your plan each week, the thumbnails are there to make it easy for you to follow along with the exercises. If you need more guidance, turn to the exercise guide (page number noted for each) to learn exactly how to do these moves. Remember to jot down any training notes as well as what weight you used for each move and each set in the space provided so you can make adjustments along the way and feel good about the progress you're making.

WEEK 2 Day 8
Full-Body Strength

WARM-UP

Perform each exercise for 30 seconds, resting 10 seconds between moves. After completing all moves, rest for one minute then repeat the circuit.

- Jumping Jack (p.131)
- Good Morning (p.130)
- Inchworm Shoulder Tap (p.116)
- Shuffle Punch (p.96)
- Knee Drive (p.117)

EXERCISE

SQUAT TO SINGLE-ARM OVERHEAD PRESS (P.139)
▶ Light to medium dumbbell

DEADLIFT AND ROW (P.136)
▶ Medium dumbbells

CURTSY LUNGE WITH BICEPS CURL (P.134)
▶ Light to medium dumbbells

DEAD CLEAN (P.133)
▶ Medium kettlebell or dumbbell

SQUAT AND SNATCH (P.137)
▶ Medium dumbbell

LOADED DEADBUG (P.114)
▶ Light dumbbells

48 Strong & Fit After 40

▶ **REST** Rest 20 seconds between each exercise and 45 seconds between sets.

WORK	SET 1	SET 2	SET 3
10 reps per side			
10 reps			
10 reps per side			
10 reps			
10 reps per side			
10 reps per side, alternating			

WEEK 2 Day 9
Upper-Body Strength

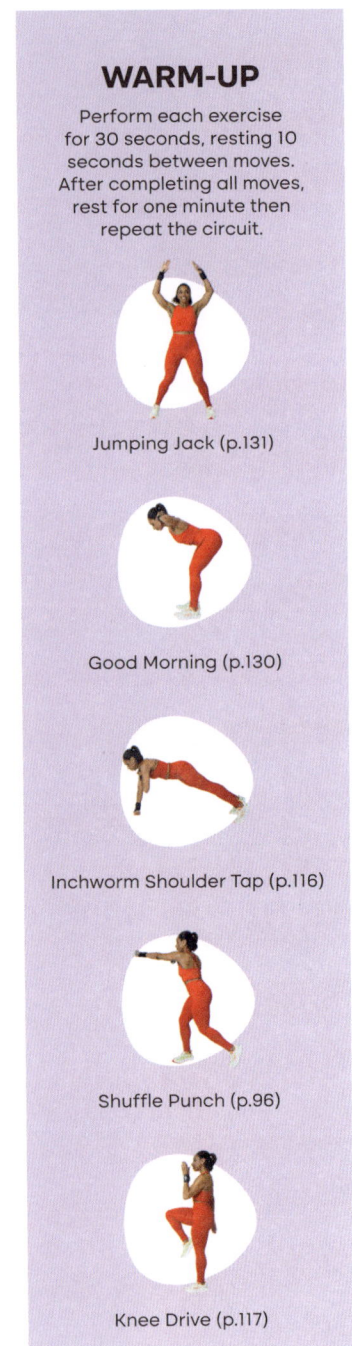

EXERCISE

WARRIOR ONE ROW (P.127)
▶ Medium dumbbells

SINGLE SINGLE DOUBLE BICEPS CURL (P.91)
▶ Light dumbbells

ISOMETRIC LATERAL RAISE (P.99)
▶ Light dumbbells

CHEST FLY (P.92)
▶ Light dumbbells

TRICEPS KICKBACK (P.94)
▶ Light dumbbells

REAR DELT FLY (P.93)
▶ Light dumbbells

▶ **REST** Rest 20 seconds between each exercise and 45 seconds between sets.

WORK	SET 1	SET 2	SET 3
10 reps per side			
10 reps			
Hold first rep 5 sec., then 10 reps more holding 5-10 sec.			
10 reps			
10 reps			
10 reps			

WEEK 2 Day 10
Rest or Active Recovery

YOUR CHOICE

Use this day to rest your body or do this active recovery routine.

EXERCISE

GOOD MORNING (P.130) ▶ Body weight	
90/90 TAP (P.112) ▶ Body weight	
DEADBUG (P.113) ▶ Body weight	
CHILD'S POSE (P.129) ▶ Body weight	
LIGHT CARDIO OF CHOICE (I.E., WALKING, CYCLING, ETC.)	

▶ **REST** Rest 30 seconds between each exercise.

WORK	SET 1
15 reps	
15 reps	
15 reps per side, alternating	
30 sec.	
10–15 min.	

GO FOR A RIDE

Whether you're pedaling outside or hopping in the saddle indoors, logging some miles on your bike can:

▼

WORK FOR ANY FITNESS LEVEL
As a non-weight bearing, low-impact activity, cycling doesn't add any extra pressure to your joints, tendons, or ligaments, making it ideal for those who are new to exercising in general, people who are injured or need rehabilitation, or people who have degenerative joints, according to *Current Sports Medicine Reports*.

▼

REDUCE THE RISK OF DISEASE
Both cycling for commuting and for exercise are consistently associated with diminished risk of type 2 diabetes. Also, people who cycle for 30 minutes five days a week take about half the sick days compared to sedentary counterparts, according to research from the University of North Carolina.

▼

BOOST JOINT HEALTH
The benefits of cycling are two-fold for your joints, according to the Arthritis Foundation. You aren't stressing your joints repeatedly, but you are also helping strengthen the muscles that support your knees, ankles, and feet.

WEEK 2 Day 11
Lower-Body Strength

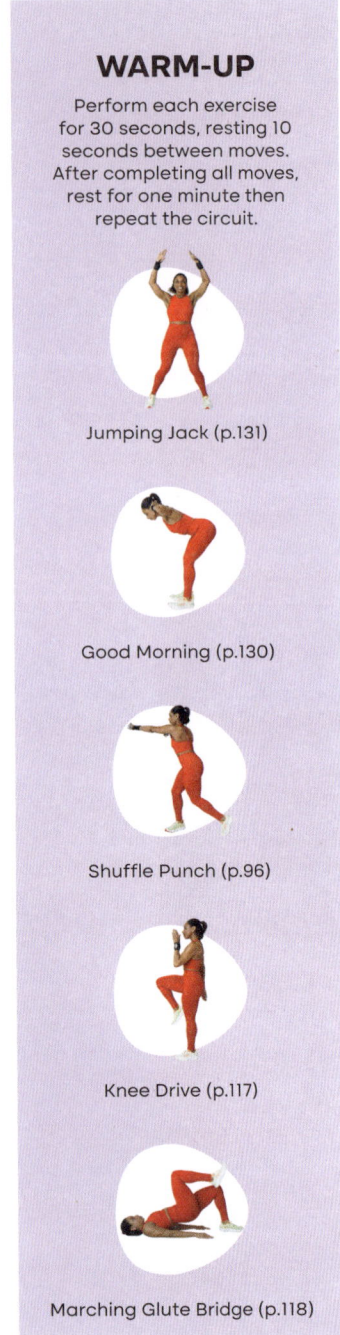

WARM-UP

Perform each exercise for 30 seconds, resting 10 seconds between moves. After completing all moves, rest for one minute then repeat the circuit.

- Jumping Jack (p.131)
- Good Morning (p.130)
- Shuffle Punch (p.96)
- Knee Drive (p.117)
- Marching Glute Bridge (p.118)

EXERCISE

REVERSE LUNGE (P.105)
▶ Medium to heavy dumbbells

DUMBBELL SUMO SQUAT (P.108)
▶ Heavy dumbbell

STAGGERED-STANCE DEADLIFT (P.103)
▶ Medium to heavy dumbbells

BANDED GLUTE BRIDGE (P.101)
▶ Medium to heavy resistance band

BANDED LATERAL STEP-OUT SQUAT (P.107)
▶ Medium resistance band

FOOTBALL SHUFFLE (P.106)
▶ Light to medium resistance band

▶ **REST** Rest 20 seconds between each exercise and 45 seconds between sets.

WORK	SET 1	SET 2	SET 3
10 reps per side			
10 reps			
10 reps per side			
12 reps			
12 reps per side			
20 sec.			

The 28-Day Plan **55**

WEEK 2 Day 12
Rest or Active Recovery

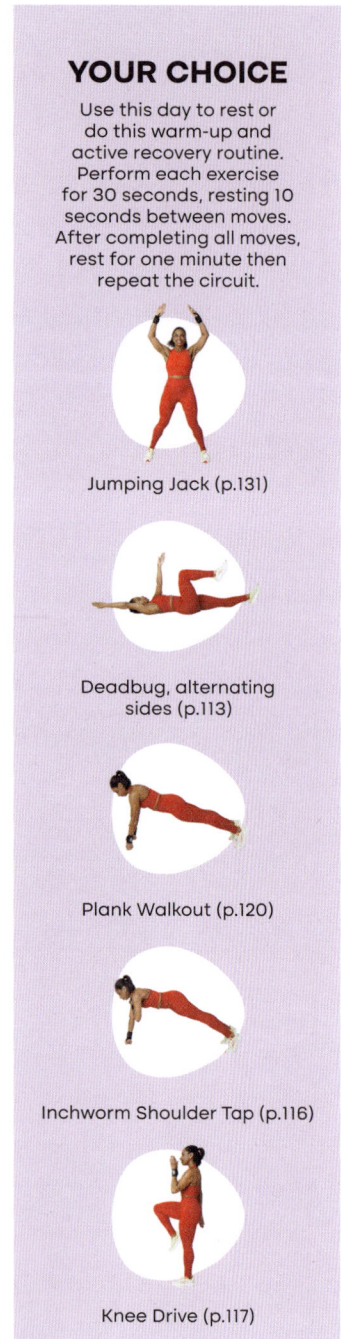

YOUR CHOICE

Use this day to rest or do this warm-up and active recovery routine. Perform each exercise for 30 seconds, resting 10 seconds between moves. After completing all moves, rest for one minute then repeat the circuit.

- Jumping Jack (p.131)
- Deadbug, alternating sides (p.113)
- Plank Walkout (p.120)
- Inchworm Shoulder Tap (p.116)
- Knee Drive (p.117)

EXERCISE

V-UP (P.126)
▶ Body weight

MOUNTAIN CLIMBER (P.119)
▶ Body weight

SCISSOR KICK (P.122)
▶ Body weight

REVERSE CRUNCH (P.121)
▶ Body weight

FARMER'S CARRY (P.115)
▶ Medium to heavy dumbbells or kettlebells

OPTIONAL LIGHT CARDIO OF CHOICE (I.E., WALKING, CYCLING, ETC.)

▶ **REST** Rest 20 seconds between each exercise and rest 45 seconds between sets.

WORK	SET 1	SET 2
15 reps		
15 reps		
15 reps		
15 reps		
20 steps		
20 min.		

WEEK 2 Day 13
Full-Body Circuit

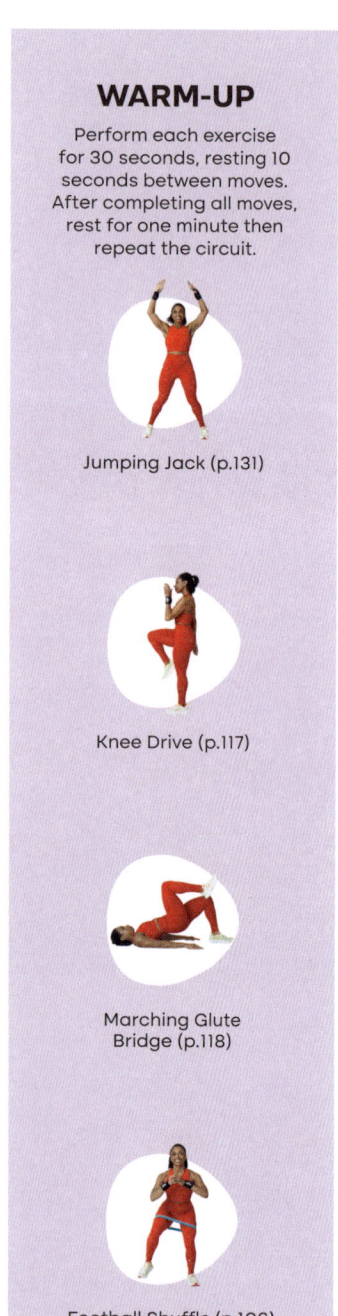

WARM-UP

Perform each exercise for 30 seconds, resting 10 seconds between moves. After completing all moves, rest for one minute then repeat the circuit.

Jumping Jack (p.131)

Knee Drive (p.117)

Marching Glute Bridge (p.118)

Football Shuffle (p.106)

EXERCISE

JUMPING JACK (P.131)
▶ Body weight

INCLINE PUSHUP (P.97)
▶ Body weight

SHUFFLE PUNCH (P.96)
▶ Body weight

FOOTBALL SHUFFLE (P.106)
▶ Body weight

JUMP SQUAT (P.109)
▶ Body weight

▶ **REST** Rest 10 seconds between each exercise and 60 seconds between sets.

WORK	SET 1	SET 2	SET 3
25 sec.			
25 sec.			
25 sec.			
25 sec.			
25 sec.			

Day 14
Rest or Light Cardio

▶ Take today off or do some light cardio, such as walking for 20 minutes, light cycling for 10 to 15 minutes, or stretching for as long as it feels good.

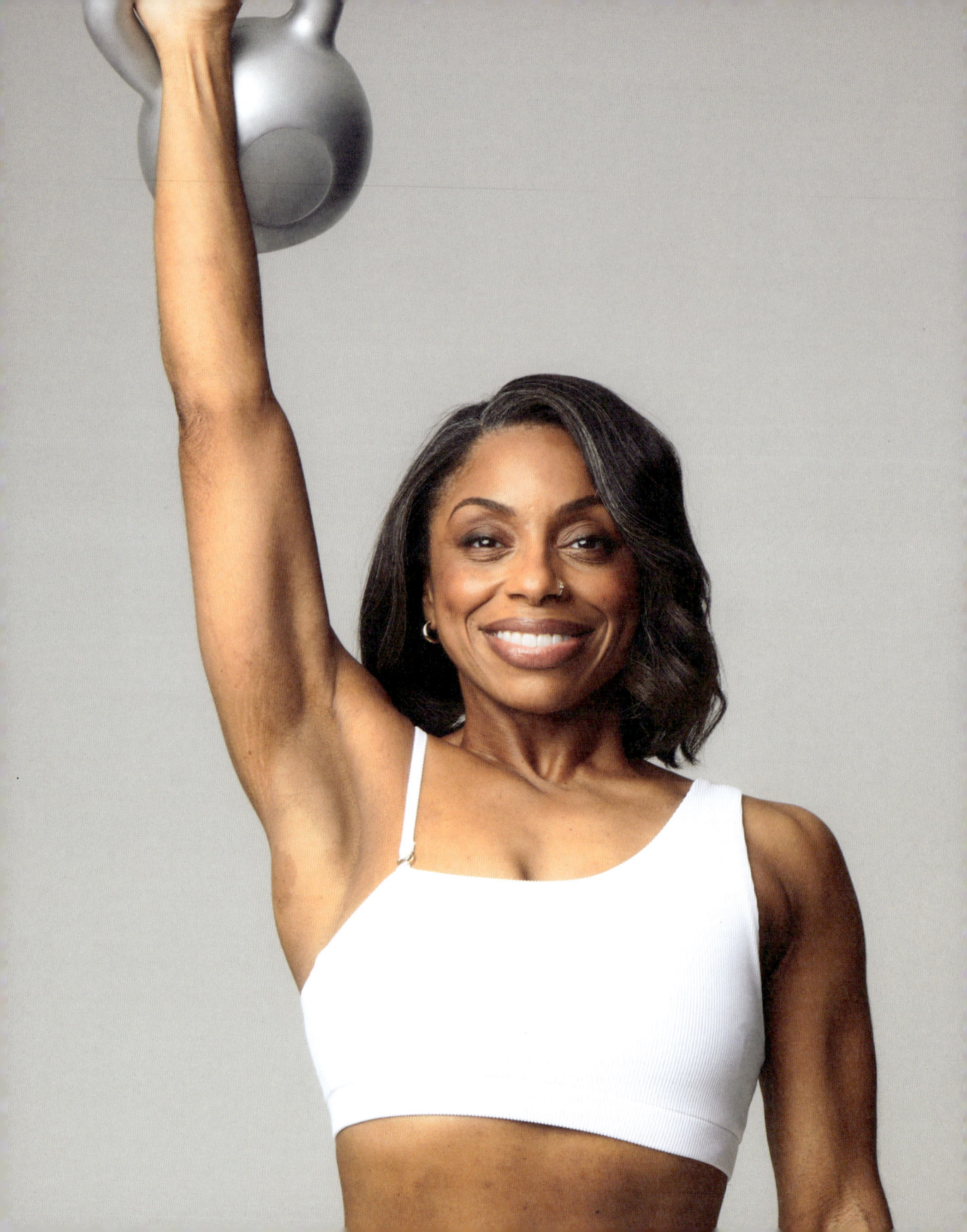

WEEK 3 At A Glance

▶ **DAY 15** Full-Body Strength

▶ **DAY 16** Upper-Body Strength

▶ **DAY 17** Active Recovery

▶ **DAY 18** Lower-Body Strength

▶ **DAY 19** Core and Stability

▶ **DAY 20** Full-Body Circuit

▶ **DAY 21** Rest or Light Cardio

TRACK YOUR PROGRESS

As you go through your plan each week, the thumbnails are there to make it easy for you to follow along with the exercises. If you need more guidance, turn to the exercise guide (page number noted for each) to learn exactly how to do these moves. Remember to jot down any training notes as well as what weight you used for each move and each set in the space provided so you can make adjustments along the way and feel good about the progress you're making.

WEEK 3 Day 15
Full-Body Strength

WARM-UP

Perform each exercise for 30 seconds, resting 10 seconds between moves. After completing all moves, rest for one minute then repeat the circuit.

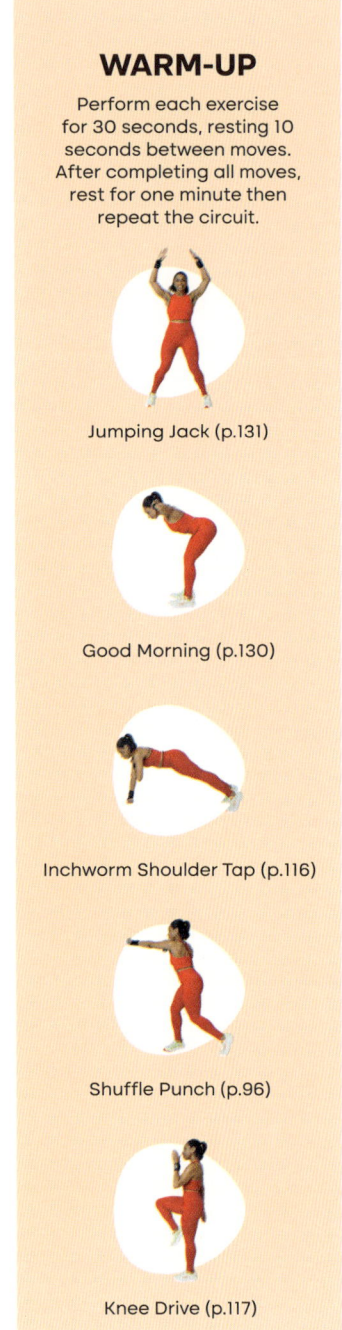

Jumping Jack (p.131)

Good Morning (p.130)

Inchworm Shoulder Tap (p.116)

Shuffle Punch (p.96)

Knee Drive (p.117)

EXERCISE

SQUAT TO OVERHEAD PRESS (P.138) ▶ Light to medium dumbbells	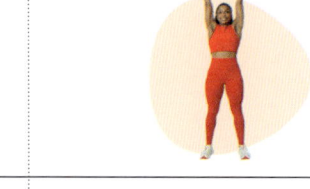
DEADLIFT AND ROW (P.136) ▶ Medium dumbbells	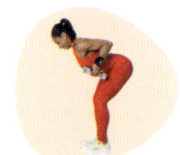
CURTSY LUNGE WITH BICEPS CURL (P.134) ▶ Light to medium dumbbells	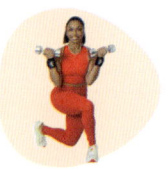
SIDE LUNGE AND ROW (P.135) ▶ Medium dumbbells	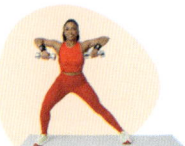
SQUAT AND SNATCH (P.137) ▶ Medium dumbbell	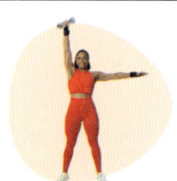
DEADBUG (P.113) ▶ Body weight	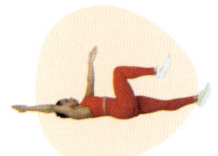

62 Strong & Fit After 40

▶ **REST** Rest 20 seconds between each exercise and 45 seconds between sets.

WORK	SET 1	SET 2	SET 3	SET 4
12 reps				
12 reps				
12 reps per side				
12 reps per side				
12 reps per side				
12 reps per side, alternating				

WEEK 3 Day 16
Upper-Body Strength

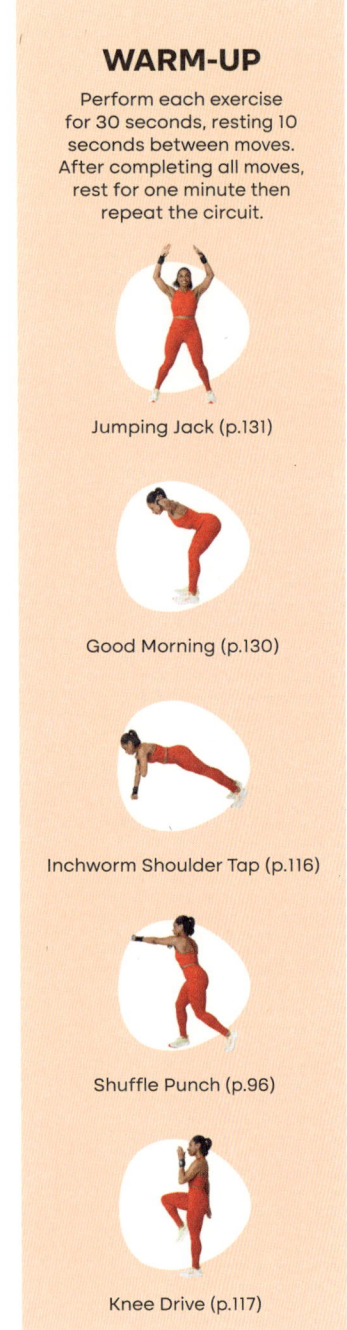

WARM-UP

Perform each exercise for 30 seconds, resting 10 seconds between moves. After completing all moves, rest for one minute then repeat the circuit.

- Jumping Jack (p.131)
- Good Morning (p.130)
- Inchworm Shoulder Tap (p.116)
- Shuffle Punch (p.96)
- Knee Drive (p.117)

EXERCISE

Exercise	
WARRIOR ONE ROW (P.127) ▶ Medium dumbbells	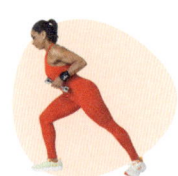
SINGLE SINGLE DOUBLE BICEPS CURL (P.91) ▶ Light dumbbells	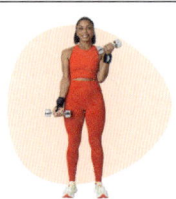
ALTERNATING FRONT AND LATERAL RAISE (P.98) ▶ Light dumbbells	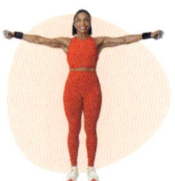
BRIDGE CHEST PRESS (P.95) ▶ Medium dumbbells	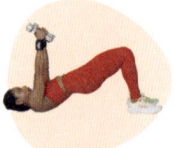
TRICEPS KICKBACK (P. 94) ▶ Light dumbbells	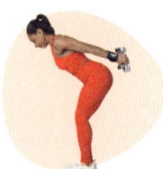
REAR DELT FLY (P.93) ▶ Light dumbbells	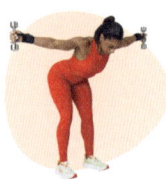

▶ **REST** Rest 20 seconds between each exercise and 45 seconds between sets.

WORK	SET 1	SET 2	SET 3	SET 4
12 reps per side				
12 reps				
12 reps				
12 reps				
12 reps				
12 reps				

The 28-Day Plan

WEEK 3 Day 17
Active Recovery

RECOVERY

Complete this active recovery routine. For an additional boost, follow the stretching routine on page 24.

EXERCISE

GOOD MORNING (P.130)
▶ Body weight

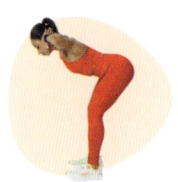

90/90 TAP (P.112)
▶ Body weight

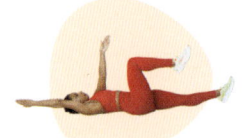

DEADBUG (P.113)
▶ Body weight

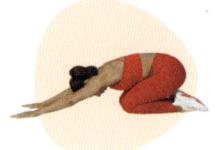

CHILD'S POSE (P.129)
▶ Body weight

LIGHT CARDIO OF CHOICE (I.E., WALKING, CYCLING, ETC.)

▶ **REST** Rest 30 seconds between each exercise and 45 to 60 seconds between sets.

WORK	SET 1	SET 2
15 reps		
15 reps		
15 reps per side, alternating		
30 sec.		
15–20 min.		

STRETCH IT OUT

When you've had a tough workout—your muscles are sore and you feel tight—pulling out a mat and running through some stretches could give your muscles and joints the relief they need.

If you have tightness in the hips and lower back, try this modification for **child's pose:**

Shweta Jain, a yoga instructor at MyYogaTeacher, suggests placing a bolster or stacked blankets lengthwise on your mat. As you lower yourself to the floor, rest your torso on the bolster or blankets.

Remember to exhale as you get into child's pose, and once holding, breathe fluidly in and out.

WEEK 3 Day 18
Lower-Body Strength

WARM-UP

Perform each exercise for 30 seconds, resting 10 seconds between moves. After completing all moves, rest for one minute then repeat the circuit.

- Jumping Jack (p.131)
- Good Morning (p.130)
- Shuffle Punch (p.96)
- Knee Drive (p.117)
- Marching Glute Bridge (p.118)

EXERCISE

REVERSE LUNGE (P.105)
▶ Medium to heavy dumbbells

DUMBBELL SUMO SQUAT (P.108)
▶ Heavy dumbbell

STAGGERED-STANCE DEADLIFT (P.103)
▶ Medium to heavy dumbbells

BANDED GLUTE BRIDGE (P.101)
▶ Medium to heavy resistance band

CLAMSHELL (P.102)
▶ Medium to heavy resistance band

FOOTBALL SHUFFLE (P.106)
▶ Light to medium resistance band

▶ **REST** Rest 20 seconds between each exercise and 45 seconds between sets.

WORK	SET 1	SET 2	SET 3	SET 4
12 reps per side				
12 reps				
12 reps per side				
15 reps				
15 reps per side				
20 sec.				

WEEK 3 Day 19
Core and Stability

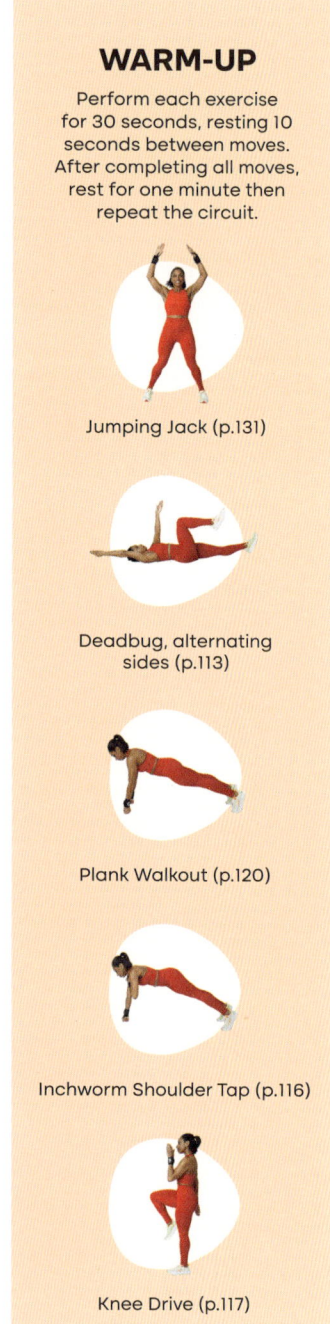

WARM-UP

Perform each exercise for 30 seconds, resting 10 seconds between moves. After completing all moves, rest for one minute then repeat the circuit.

- Jumping Jack (p.131)
- Deadbug, alternating sides (p.113)
- Plank Walkout (p.120)
- Inchworm Shoulder Tap (p.116)
- Knee Drive (p.117)

EXERCISE

V-UP (P.126)
▶ Body weight

MOUNTAIN CLIMBER (P.119)
▶ Body weight

SCISSOR KICK (P.122)
▶ Body weight

SUPERMAN (P.123)
▶ Body weight

FARMER'S CARRY (P.115)
▶ Medium to heavy dumbbells or kettlebells

MODIFIED BURPEE (P.132)
▶ Light dumbbells

▶ **REST** Rest 20 seconds between each exercise and 45 seconds between sets.

WORK	SET 1	SET 2	SET 3
15 reps			
15 reps			
15 reps			
15 reps			
20 steps			
10 reps			

The 28-Day Plan

WEEK 3 Day 20
Full-Body Circuit

WARM-UP

Perform each exercise for 30 seconds, resting 10 seconds between moves. After completing all moves, rest for one minute then repeat the circuit.

- Jumping Jack (p.131)
- Knee Drive (p.117)
- Marching Glute Bridge (p.118)
- Football Shuffle (p.106)

EXERCISE	WORK
JUMPING JACK (P.131) ▶ Body weight	30 sec.
INCLINE PUSHUP (P.97) ▶ Body weight	30 sec.
SHUFFLE PUNCH (P.96) ▶ Body weight	30 sec.
FOOTBALL SHUFFLE (P.106) ▶ Body weight	30 sec.
JUMP SQUAT (P.109) ▶ Body weight	30 sec.

Strong & Fit After 40

▶ **REST** Rest 10 seconds between each exercise and 60 seconds between sets.

SET 1	SET 2	SET 3	SET 4

Day 21
Rest or Light Cardio

▶ Take today off or do some light cardio, such as walking for 20 minutes, light cycling for 10 to 15 minutes, or stretching for as long as it feels good.

The 28-Day Plan

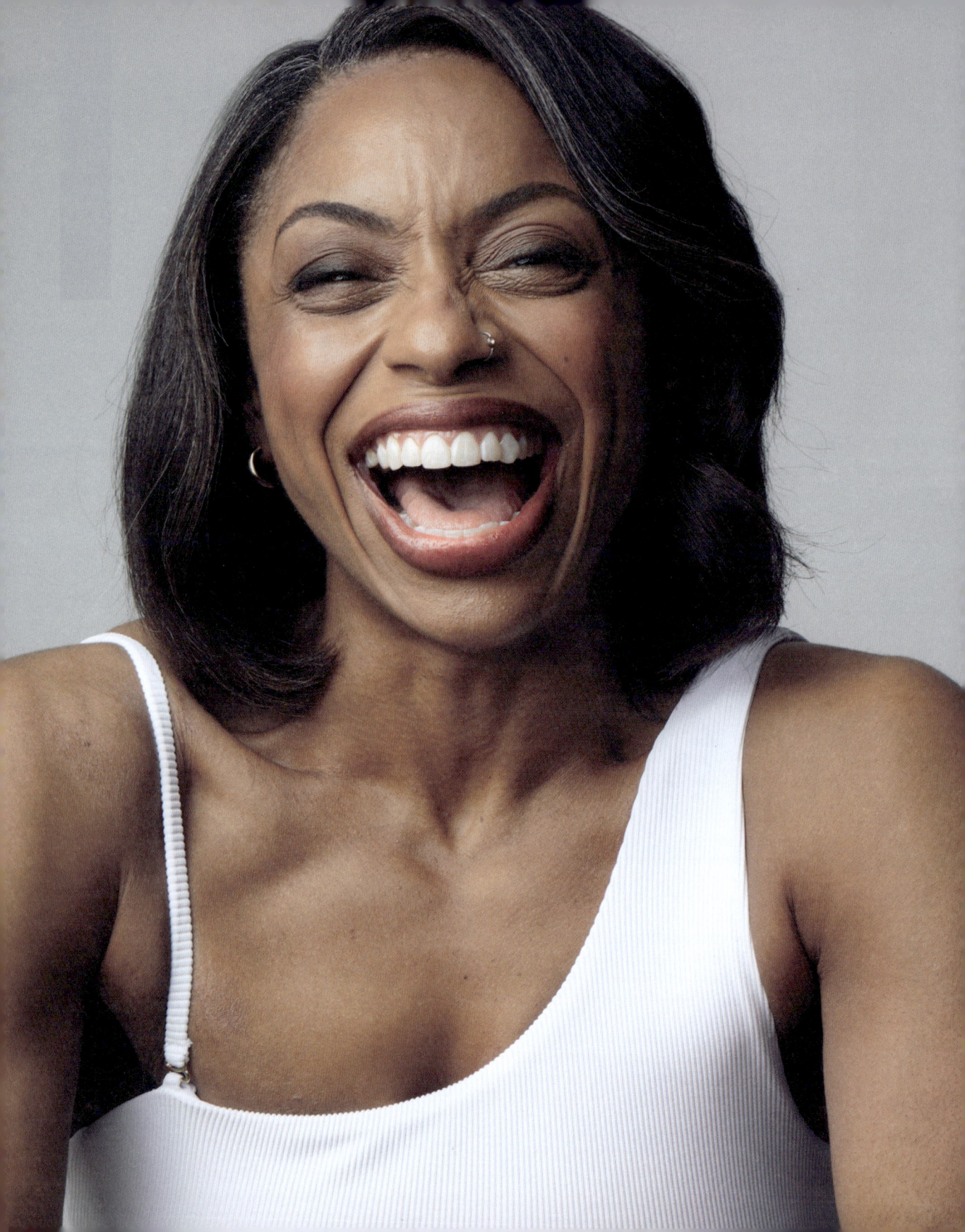

WEEK 4 At A Glance

▶ **DAY 22** Full-Body Strength

▶ **DAY 23** Upper-Body Strength

▶ **DAY 24** Active Recovery

▶ **DAY 25** Lower-Body Strength

▶ **DAY 26** Core and Stability

▶ **DAY 27** Full-Body Circuit

▶ **DAY 28** Rest or Light Cardio

TRACK YOUR PROGRESS

As you go through your plan each week, the thumbnails are there to make it easy for you to follow along with the exercises. If you need more guidance, turn to the exercise guide (page number noted for each) to learn exactly how to do these moves. Remember to jot down any training notes as well as what weight you used for each move and each set in the space provided so you can make adjustments along the way and feel good about the progress you're making.

WEEK 4 Day 22
Full-Body Strength

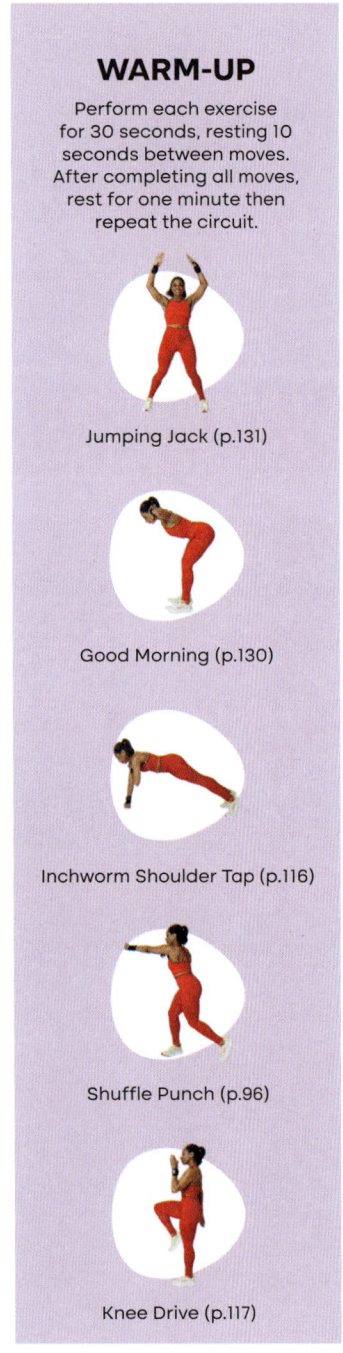

WARM-UP

Perform each exercise for 30 seconds, resting 10 seconds between moves. After completing all moves, rest for one minute then repeat the circuit.

- Jumping Jack (p.131)
- Good Morning (p.130)
- Inchworm Shoulder Tap (p.116)
- Shuffle Punch (p.96)
- Knee Drive (p.117)

EXERCISE

SQUAT TO SINGLE-ARM OVERHEAD PRESS (P.139)
▶ Light to medium dumbbell

DEADLIFT AND ROW (P.136)
▶ Medium to heavy dumbbells

CURTSY LUNGE WITH BICEPS CURL (P.134)
▶ Light to medium dumbbells

DEAD CLEAN (P.133)
▶ Medium kettlebell or dumbbell

SQUAT AND SNATCH (P.137)
▶ Medium dumbbell

LOADED DEADBUG (P.114)
▶ Light dumbbells

▶ **REST** Rest 20 seconds between each exercise and 45 seconds between sets.

WORK	SET 1	SET 2	SET 3	SET 4
12 reps per side				
12 reps				
12 reps per side				
12 reps				
12 reps per side				
12 reps per side, alternating				

WEEK 4 Day 23
Upper-Body Strength

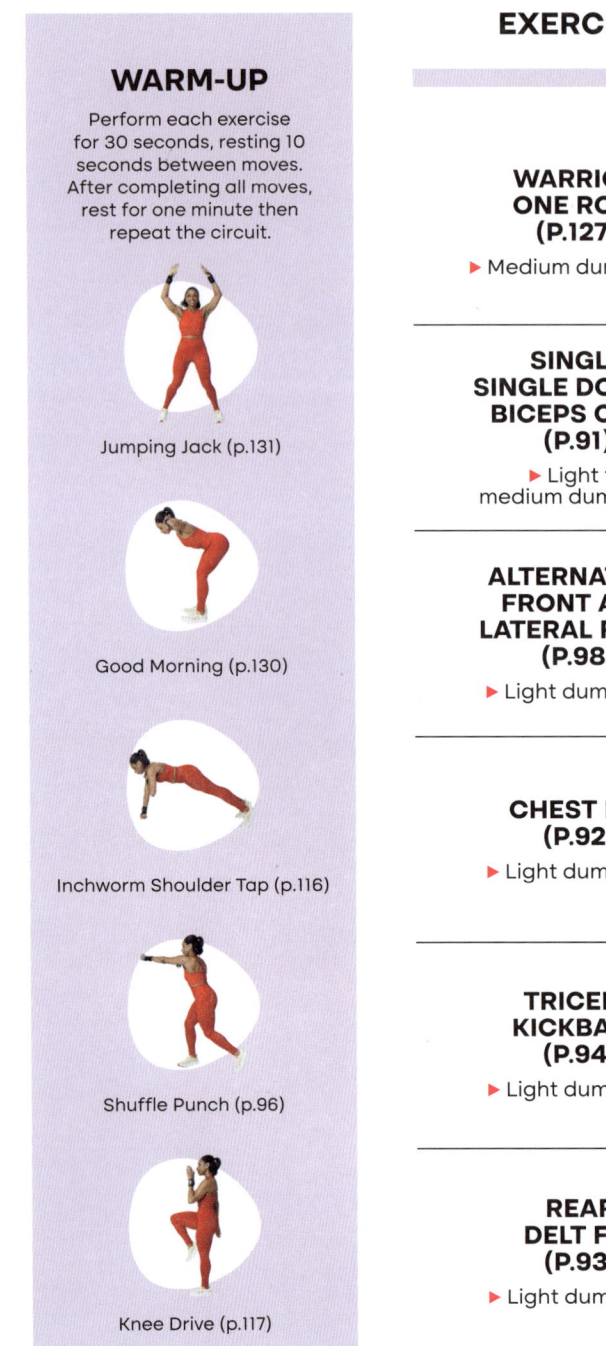

WARM-UP

Perform each exercise for 30 seconds, resting 10 seconds between moves. After completing all moves, rest for one minute then repeat the circuit.

- Jumping Jack (p.131)
- Good Morning (p.130)
- Inchworm Shoulder Tap (p.116)
- Shuffle Punch (p.96)
- Knee Drive (p.117)

EXERCISE

WARRIOR ONE ROW (P.127)
▶ Medium dumbbells

SINGLE SINGLE DOUBLE BICEPS CURL (P.91)
▶ Light to medium dumbbells

ALTERNATING FRONT AND LATERAL RAISE (P.98)
▶ Light dumbbells

CHEST FLY (P.92)
▶ Light dumbbells

TRICEPS KICKBACK (P.94)
▶ Light dumbbells

REAR DELT FLY (P.93)
▶ Light dumbbells

▶ **REST** Rest 20 seconds between each exercise and 45 seconds between sets.

WORK	SET 1	SET 2	SET 3	SET 4
12 reps per side				
12 reps				
12 reps				
12 reps				
12 reps				
12 reps				

WEEK 4 Day 24
Active Recovery

RECOVERY
Complete this active recovery routine. For an additional boost, follow the stretching routine on page 24.

EXERCISE

GOOD MORNING (P.130)
▶ Body weight

90/90 TAP (P.112)
▶ Body weight

DEADBUG (P. 113)
▶ Body weight

CHILD'S POSE (P.129)
▶ Body weight

LIGHT CARDIO OF CHOICE (I.E., WALKING, CYCLING, ETC.)

▶ **REST** Rest 30 seconds between each exercise and 45 to 60 seconds between sets.

WORK	SET 1	SET 2	SET 3
15 reps			
15 reps			
15 reps per side, alternating			
30 sec.			
20–25 min.			

The 28-Day Plan **81**

WEEK 4 Day 25
Lower-Body Strength

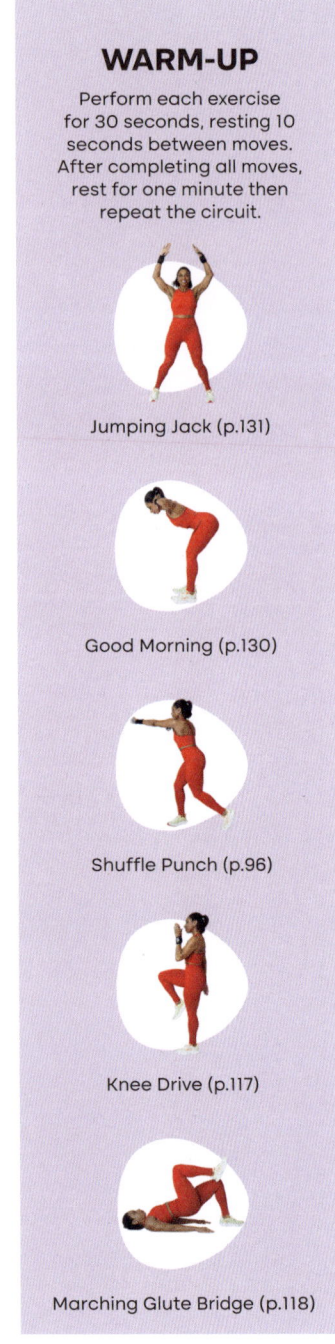

WARM-UP

Perform each exercise for 30 seconds, resting 10 seconds between moves. After completing all moves, rest for one minute then repeat the circuit.

- Jumping Jack (p.131)
- Good Morning (p.130)
- Shuffle Punch (p.96)
- Knee Drive (p.117)
- Marching Glute Bridge (p.118)

EXERCISE

REVERSE LUNGE (P.105)
▶ Medium to heavy dumbbells

DUMBBELL SUMO SQUAT (P.108)
▶ Heavy dumbbell

STAGGERED-STANCE DEADLIFT (P.103)
▶ Medium to heavy dumbbells

BANDED GLUTE BRIDGE (P.101)
▶ Medium to heavy resistance band

BANDED LATERAL STEP-OUT SQUAT (P.107)
▶ Medium resistance band

FOOTBALL SHUFFLE (P.106)
▶ Light to medium resistance band

82 Strong & Fit After 40

▶ **REST** Rest 20 seconds between each exercise and 45 seconds between sets.

WORK	SET 1	SET 2	SET 3	SET 4
12 reps per side				
12 reps				
12 reps per side				
15 reps				
15 reps per side				
25 sec.				

WEEK 4 Day 26
Core and Stability

WARM-UP

Perform each exercise for 30 seconds, resting 10 seconds between moves. After completing all moves, rest for one minute then repeat the circuit.

- Jumping Jack (p.131)
- Deadbug, alternating sides (p.113)
- Plank Walkout (p.120)
- Inchworm Shoulder Tap (p.116)
- Knee Drive (p.117)

EXERCISE

V-UP (P.126)
- Body weight

MOUNTAIN CLIMBER (P.119)
- Body weight

SCISSOR KICK (P.122)
- Body weight

REVERSE CRUNCH (P.121)
- Body weight

FARMER'S CARRY (P.115)
- Medium to heavy dumbbells or kettlebells

MODIFIED BURPEE (P.132)
- Light dumbbells

84 Strong & Fit After 40

▶ **REST** Rest 20 seconds between each exercise and 45 seconds between sets.

WORK	SET 1	SET 2	SET 3	SET 4
15 reps				
15 reps				
15 reps				
15 reps				
20 steps				
15 reps				

The 28-Day Plan

WEEK 4 Day 27
Full-Body Circuit

WARM-UP

Perform each exercise for 30 seconds, resting 10 seconds between moves. After completing all moves, rest for one minute then repeat the circuit.

- Jumping Jack (p.131)
- Knee Drive (p.117)
- Marching Glute Bridge (p.118)
- Football Shuffle (p.106)

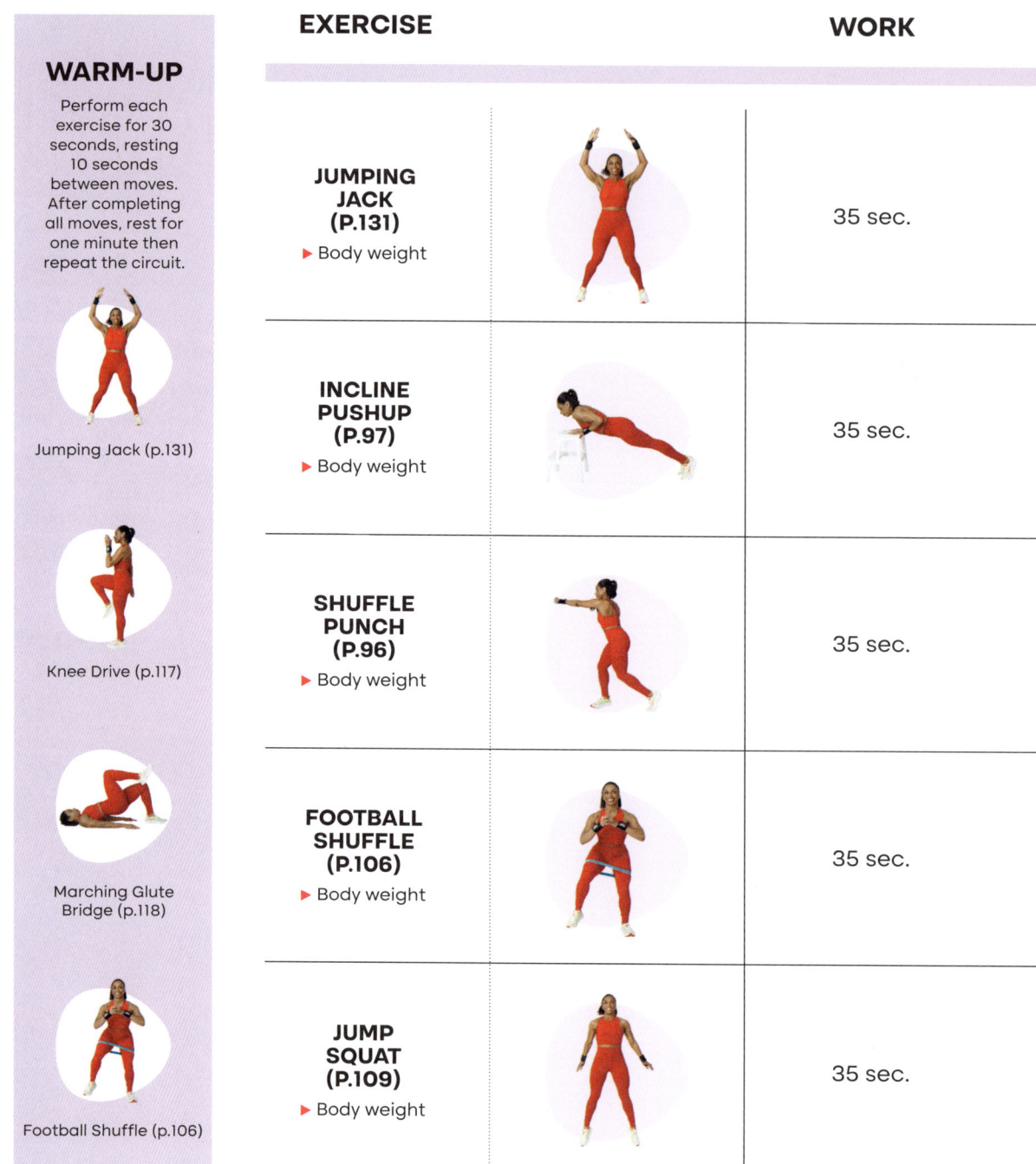

EXERCISE	WORK
JUMPING JACK (P.131) ▶ Body weight	35 sec.
INCLINE PUSHUP (P.97) ▶ Body weight	35 sec.
SHUFFLE PUNCH (P.96) ▶ Body weight	35 sec.
FOOTBALL SHUFFLE (P.106) ▶ Body weight	35 sec.
JUMP SQUAT (P.109) ▶ Body weight	35 sec.

86 Strong & Fit After 40

▶ **REST** Rest 20 seconds between each exercise and 90 seconds between sets.

SET 1	SET 2	SET 3	SET 4

Day 28
Rest or Light Cardio

▶ Take today off or do some light cardio, such as walking for 20 minutes, light cycling for 10 to 15 minutes, or stretching for as long as it feels good.

CHAPTER 4

Exercise Guide

Upper Body

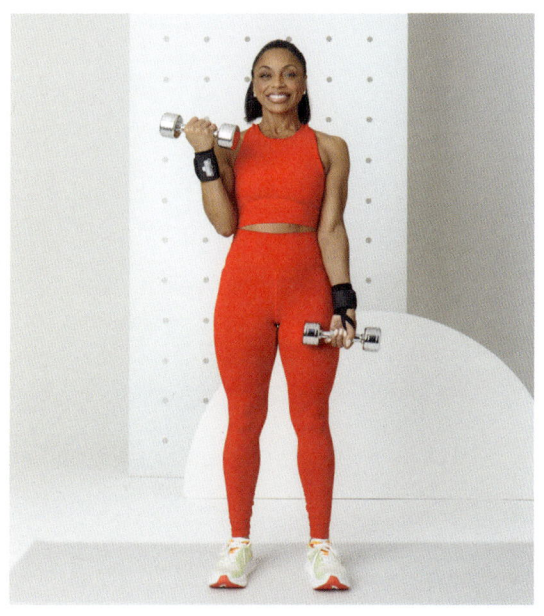
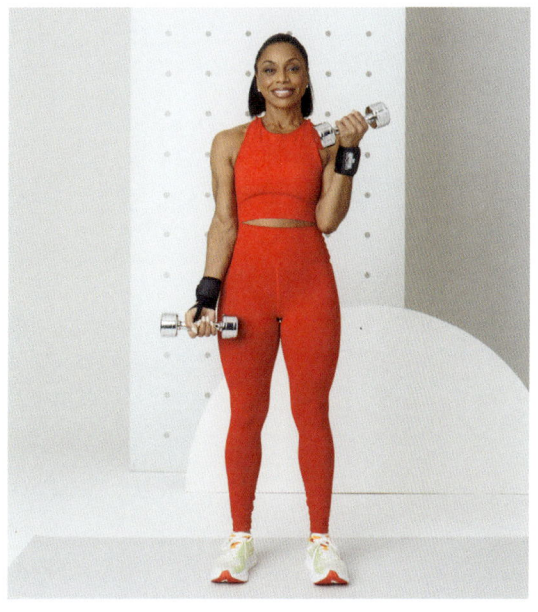
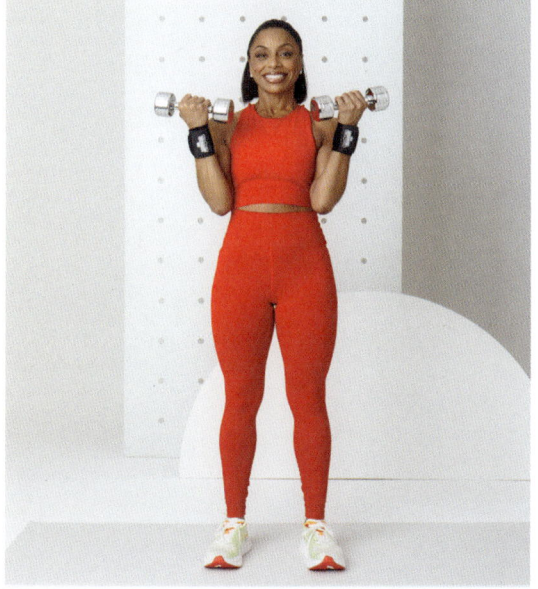

Single Single Double Biceps Curl

▶ Start standing with feet hip-width apart, one dumbbell in each hand, palms facing front. Core and glutes engaged, raise dumbbell in right hand to right shoulder. Lower it back down.

▶ Repeat with the left side. Lower left hand back down.

▶ Then perform a biceps curl with both arms simultaneously. Lower back down. That's 1 rep.

EXERCISE GUIDE Upper Body

Chest Fly

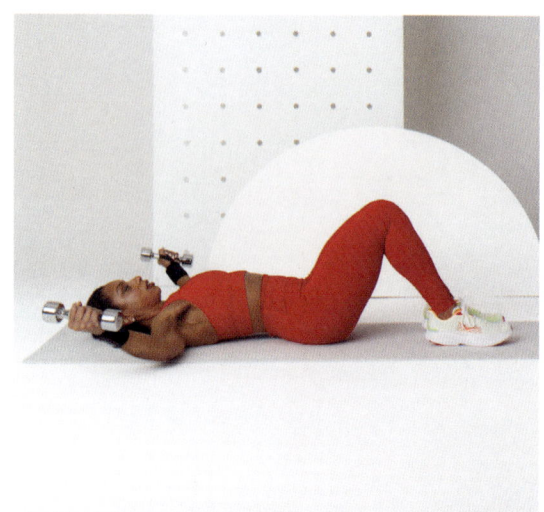

▶ Lie faceup with knees bent and feet flat on floor. Grasp dumbbells with palms facing inward.

▶ Push dumbbells directly above chest with lightly bent elbows, keeping wrists straight. Inhale and slowly lower dumbbells out to sides toward floor at shoulder height maintaining a soft roundness with your arms (think: hugging a tree).

▶ Stop when back of upper arms touch mat. Exhale and slowly raise dumbbells back to the starting position while maintaining arc in your arms. That's 1 rep.

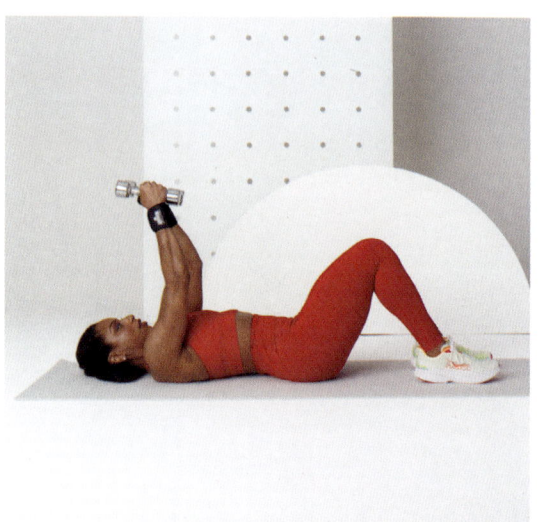

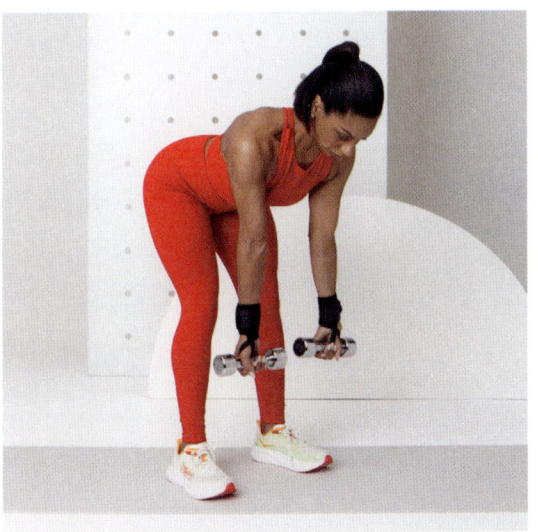
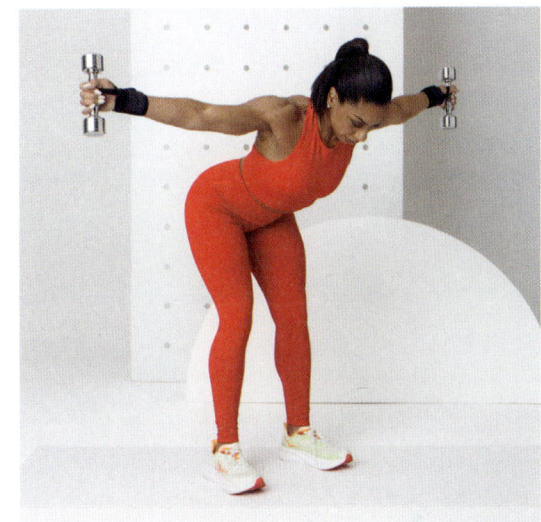

Rear Delt Fly

▶ Stand with feet hip-width apart, holding dumbbells with palms facing forward.

▶ Hinge at hips until chest is parallel to floor.

▶ Raise arms out to sides until they reach shoulder height or higher. Keep wrists neutral and thumbs up. Reverse to return to start. That's 1 rep.

EXERCISE GUIDE Upper Body

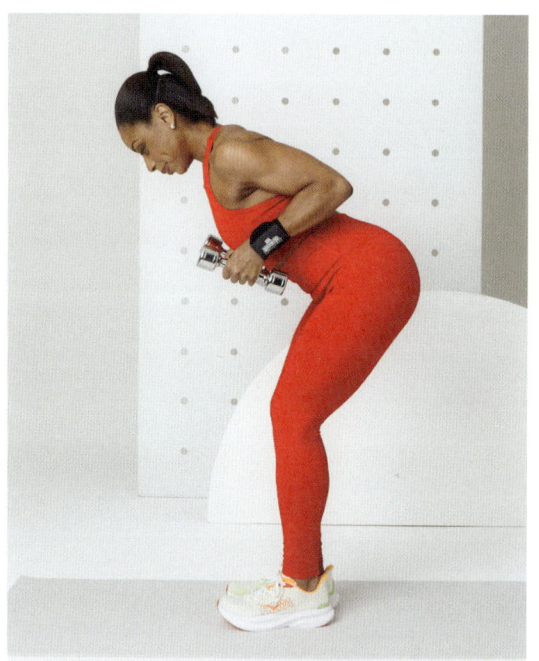 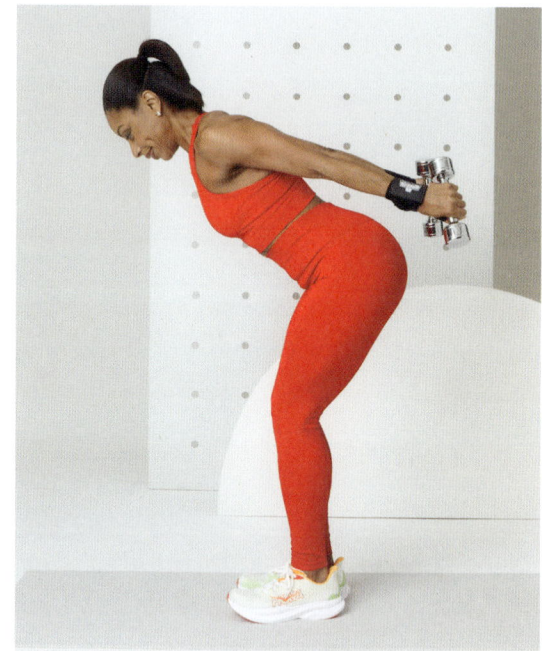

Triceps Kickback

- Start standing with feet two-fists-width apart with knees bent. Lean forward slightly, with a dumbbell in each hand and elbows at 90 degrees by sides.
- Press dumbbells back and up, and as you straighten arms, squeeze triceps. Lower weights with control to return to start. That's 1 rep.

Bridge Chest Press

▶ Lie faceup on floor with knees bent and feet flat on floor. With a dumbbell in each hand, extend arms directly over shoulders, palms facing inward. Squeeze glutes to press hips off floor until torso forms straight line.

▶ Squeeze shoulder blades together and slowly bend elbows, lowering weights down to hips, in-line with shoulders, until elbows form 90-degree angles.

▶ Slowly drive dumbbells back up to start, squeezing shoulder blades the entire time. That's 1 rep.

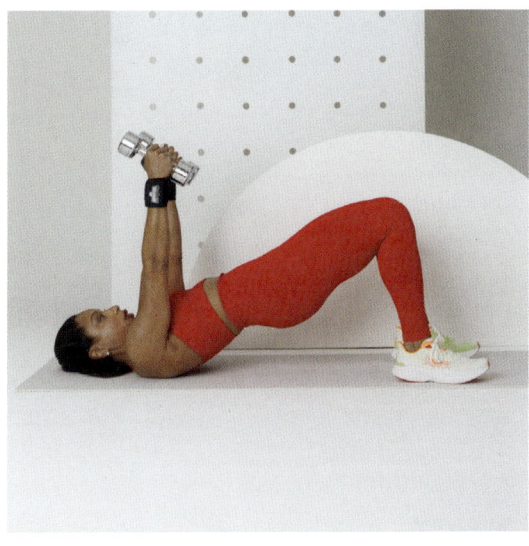

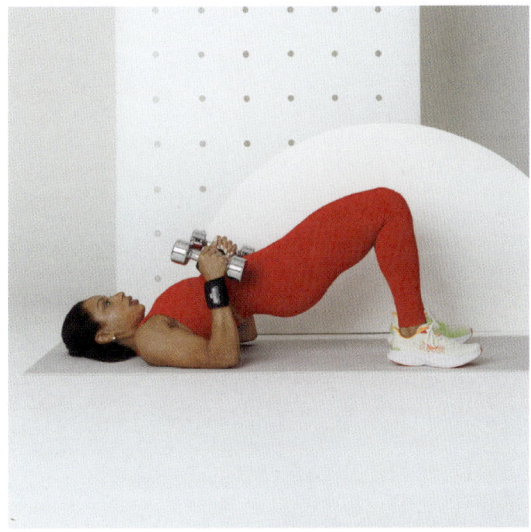

EXERCISE GUIDE Upper Body

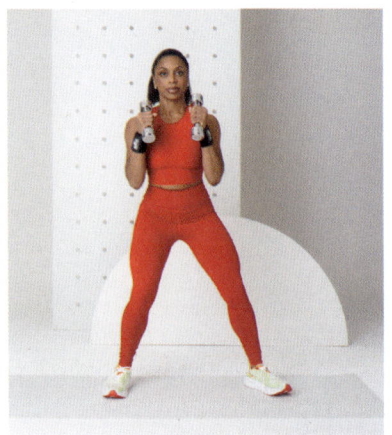
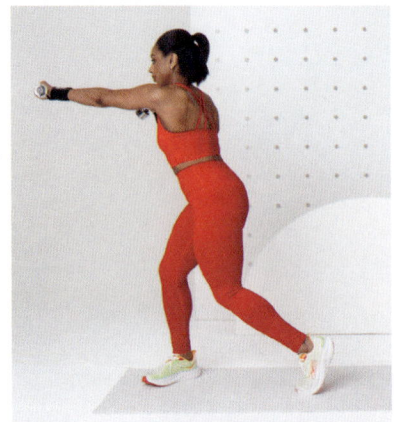
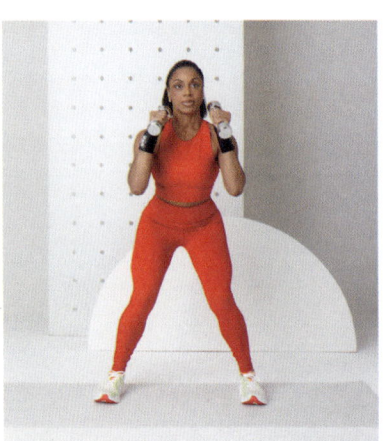
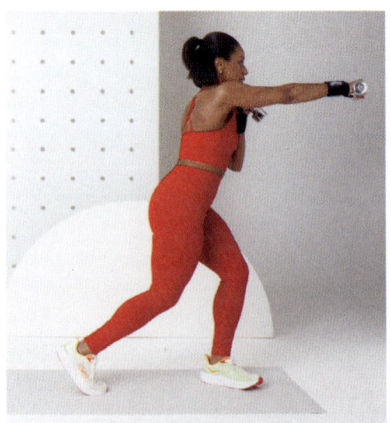

Shuffle Punch

▶ Holding a pair of dumbbells at shoulder height, quickly shuffle to the right, then pivot feet and punch left arm across body.

▶ Reverse motion to return to start.

▶ Repeat on other side. Perform for prescribed amount of time.

MODIFY IT: Perform the exercise as described above but without weights.

Incline Pushup

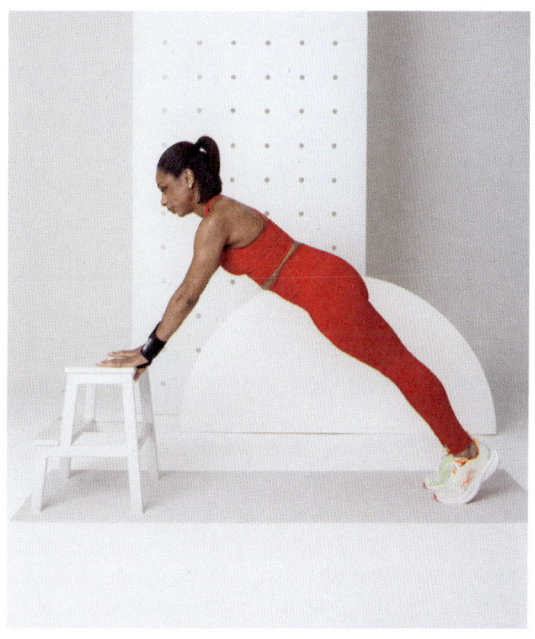

▶ Start in high plank position, with hands on an elevated surface and feet more than hip-width apart for greater stability. Think about wrapping your shoulders back, keeping your ribcage knit together, and engaging your core. (Option to start on knees or in full plank on a flat surface depending on your current strength.)

▶ With control, bend elbows and lower chest as low as you can. Push into your entire hand and press yourself back up. That's 1 rep; perform for prescribed number of reps or amount of time.

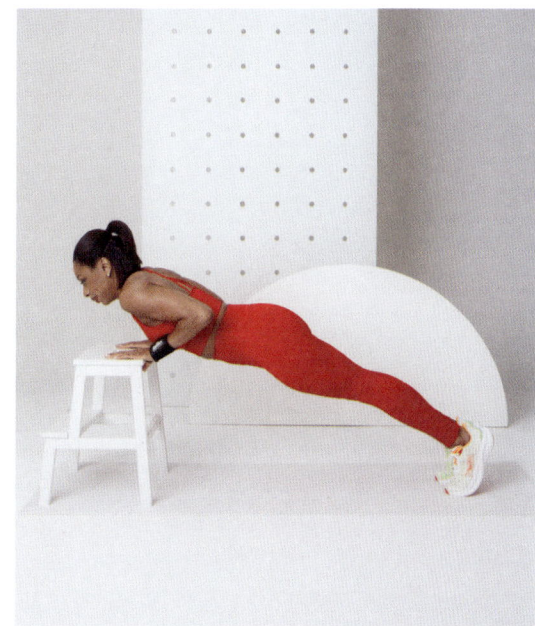

EXERCISE GUIDE Upper Body

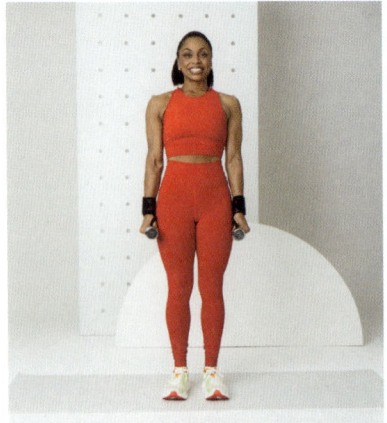
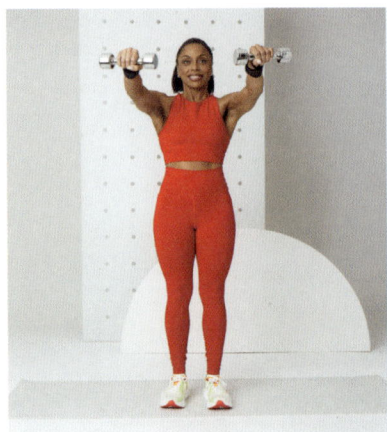
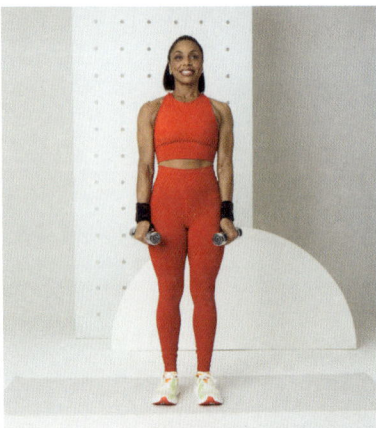
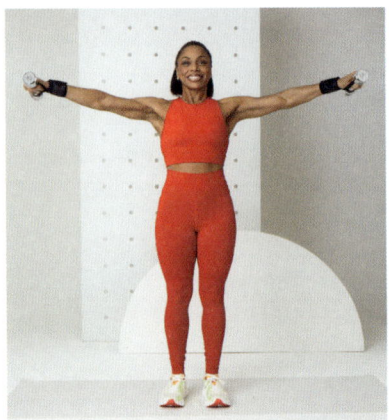

Alternating Front and Lateral Raise

▶ Stand with knees slightly bent, feet hip-width apart, and arms down by sides, holding dumbbells in each hand.

▶ Raise arms in front until hands reach shoulder height. Lower arms with control to sides.

▶ Raise arms out to sides until hands reach shoulder height. Lower arms slowly to return to start. That's 1 rep.

Isometric Lateral Raise

▶ Hold a light dumbbell in each hand and stand with feet shoulder-width apart, arms hanging straight down at your sides, palms facing in.

▶ Slowly raise arms out to sides until hands reach shoulder height. Hold for 5 to 10 seconds, then return to start. That's 1 rep.

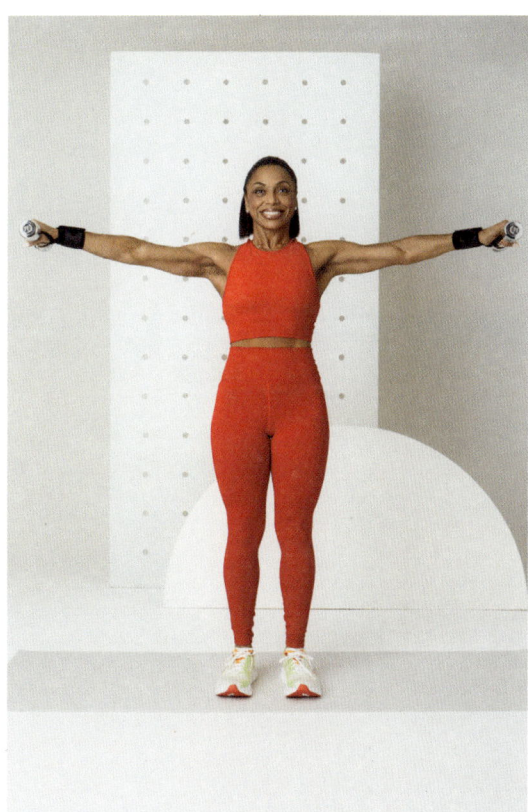

Lower Body

Banded Glute Bridge

▶ Place a miniband around thighs and lie faceup with feet flat on floor and knees bent. Squeeze glutes and lift hips off floor until body forms a straight line from knees to shoulders.

▶ Pause at the top, then lower back down to starting position. That's 1 rep.

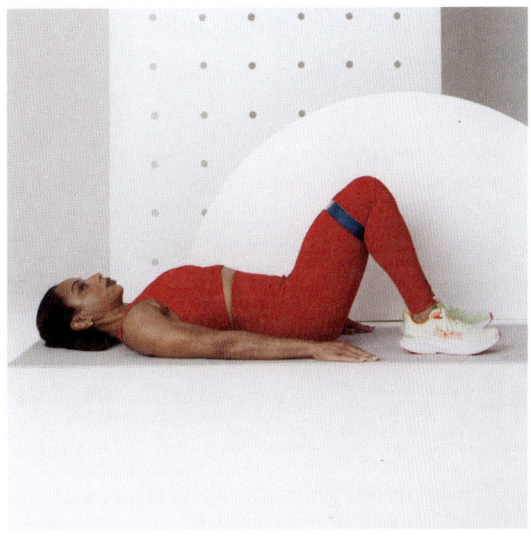

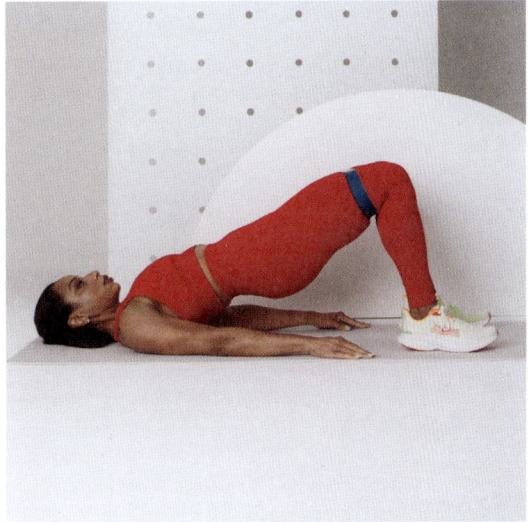

EXERCISE GUIDE Lower Body

Clamshell

▶ Start lying on right side with resistance band wrapped around thighs and upper body propped on right forearm.

▶ Bend legs so knees face forward while feet line up with glutes. Keep hips and feet still while lifting top knee as far as you can toward ceiling, then lower back to start. That's 1 rep.

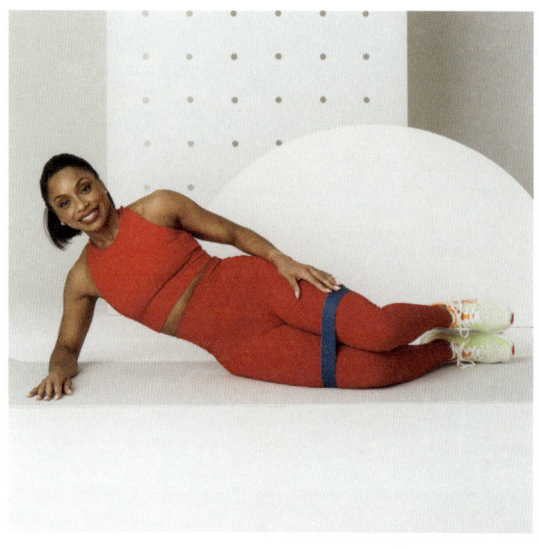

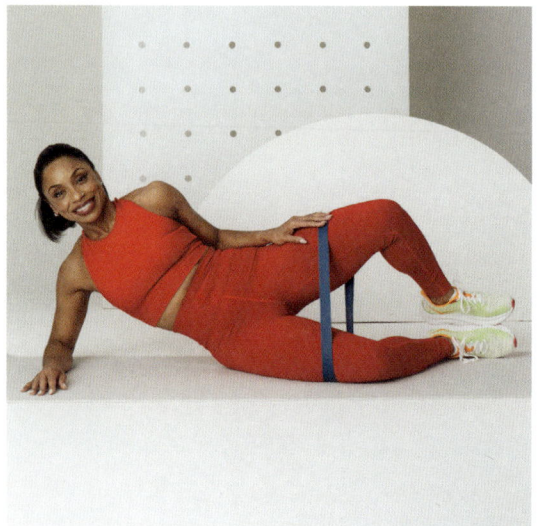

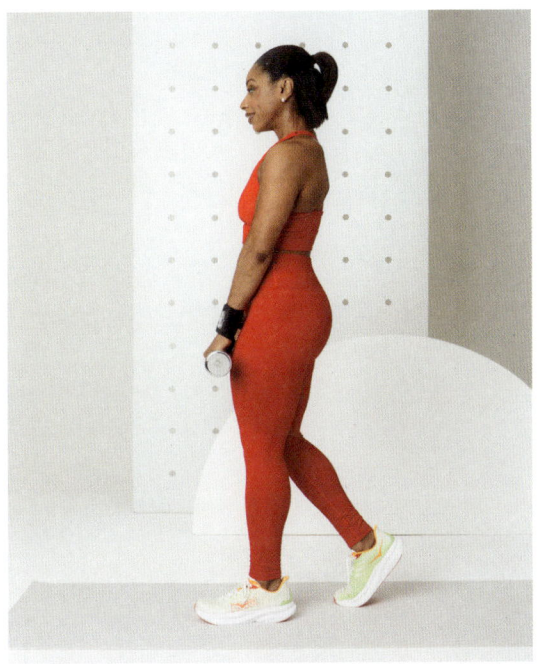
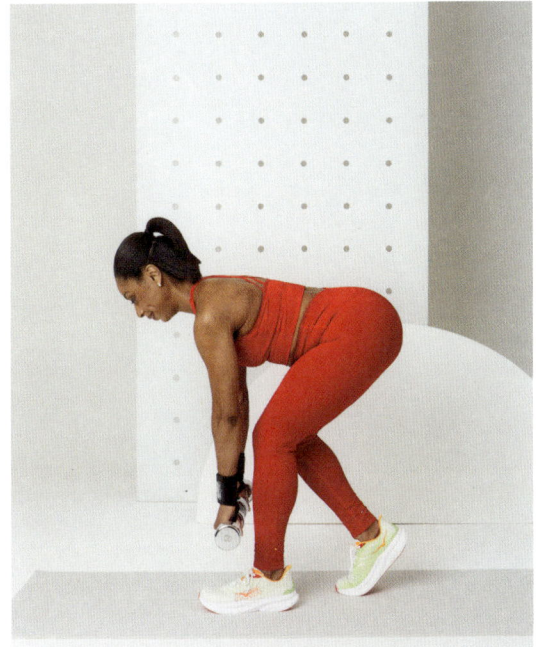

Staggered-Stance Deadlift

▶ Stand with feet hip-width apart, holding one dumbbell in each hand with palms facing legs. Then move right foot back so toes are slightly behind left heel (most of your weight should be on the left foot). Keeping spine long, send hips back as you hinge at waist.

▶ Lower weights to shin, or as far as you can without curving spine. Pause, then reverse, engaging glutes and core at top. That's 1 rep.

EXERCISE GUIDE Lower Body

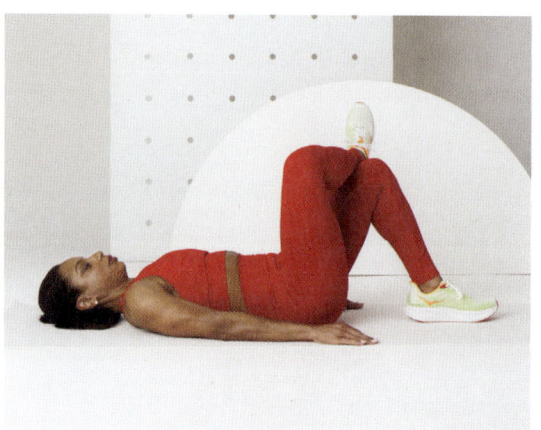 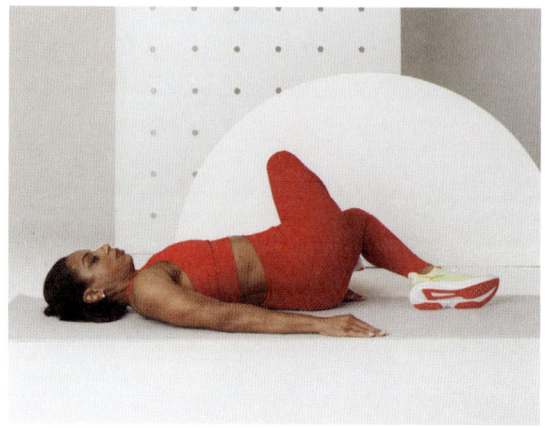

Figure Four to Twist

▶ Lie faceup with both legs bent, right ankle over left knee. Allow legs to fall to the left and hold for prescribed amount of time. Repeat on other side.

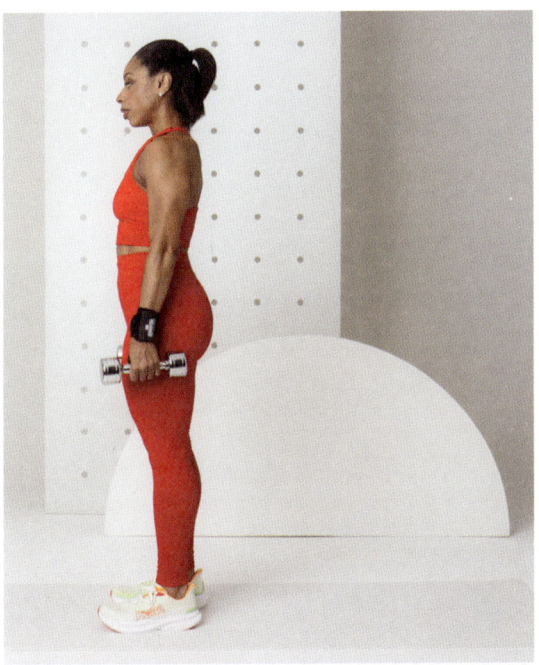
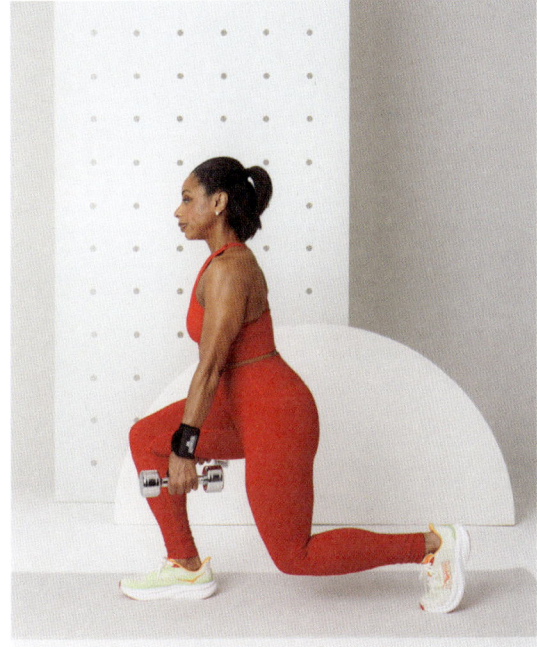

Reverse Lunge

- Start standing tall with feet directly beneath hips and arms at sides, holding dumbbells.
- Engage core and take a big step back with left foot. Keeping front knee in line with front foot, bend both legs until back knee taps floor directly beneath hip.
- Push through feet to reverse movement and return to start. That's 1 rep.

EXERCISE GUIDE Lower Body

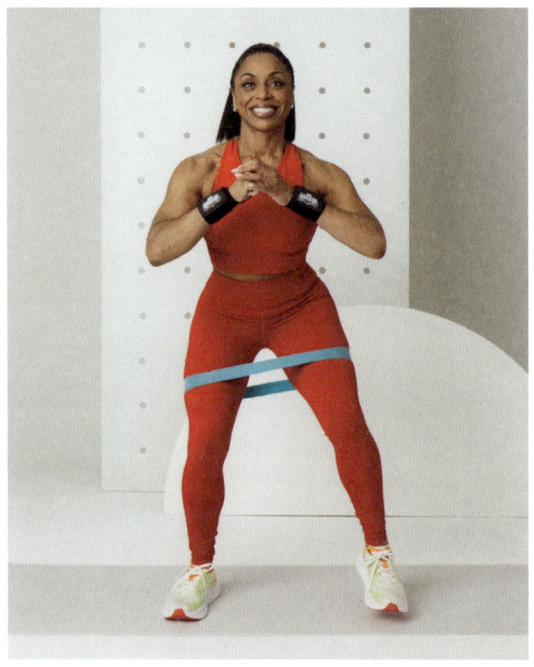

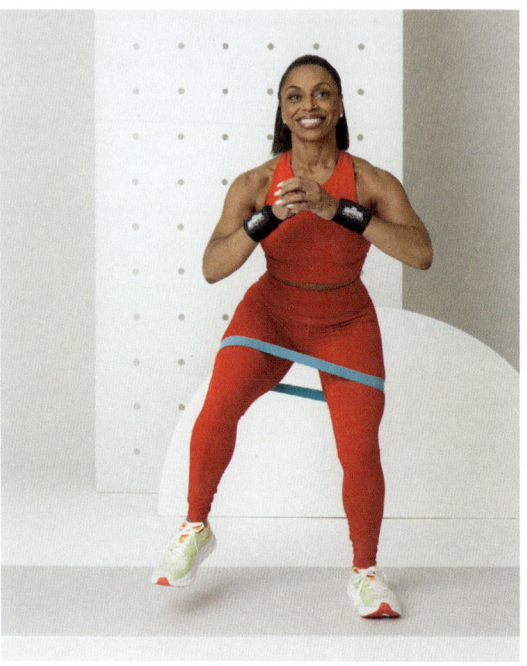

Football Shuffle

▶ With band around thighs, start standing with feet more than hip-width apart, torso slightly hinged forward.

▶ Run in place as quickly as you can while keeping tension on band for prescribed amount of time.

MODIFY IT: Perform the exercise as described above but without a resistance band.

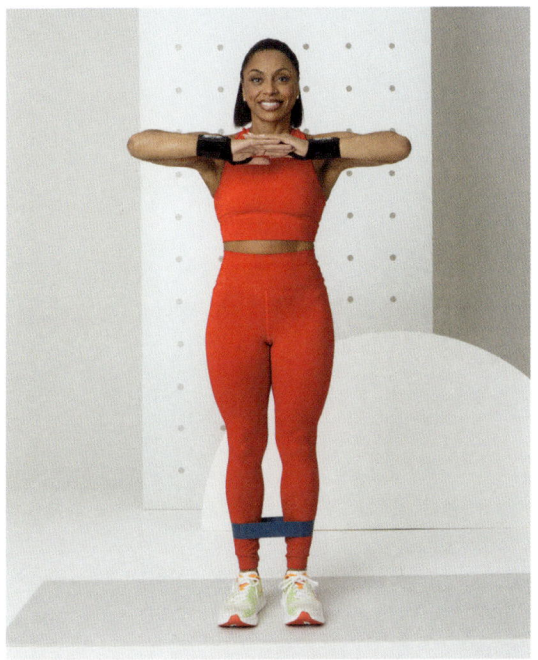
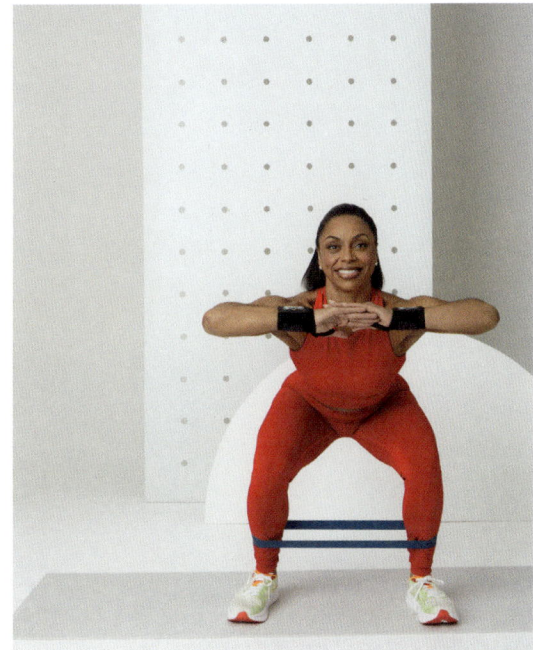

Banded Lateral Step-Out Squat

▶ Start standing with a resistance band wrapped just below knees, feet under hips, and hands clasped in front of chest.

▶ Take a big step to the left, then bend knees, sit back, and lower until thighs are parallel to floor.

▶ Engage glutes and press back up through heels to starting position. That's 1 rep.

EXERCISE GUIDE Lower Body

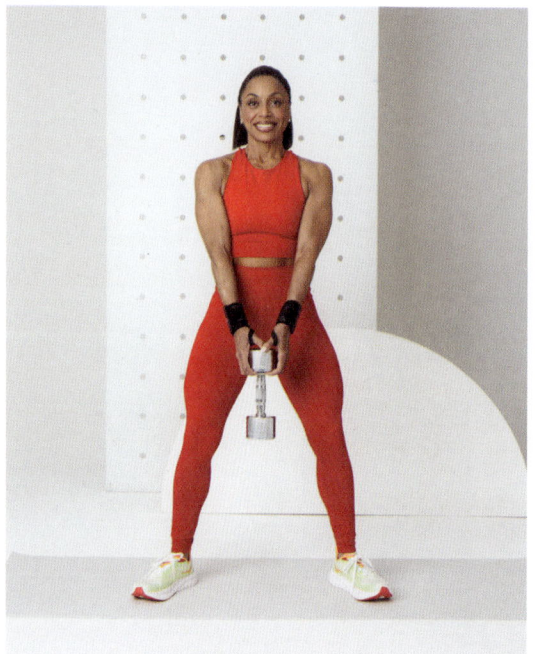 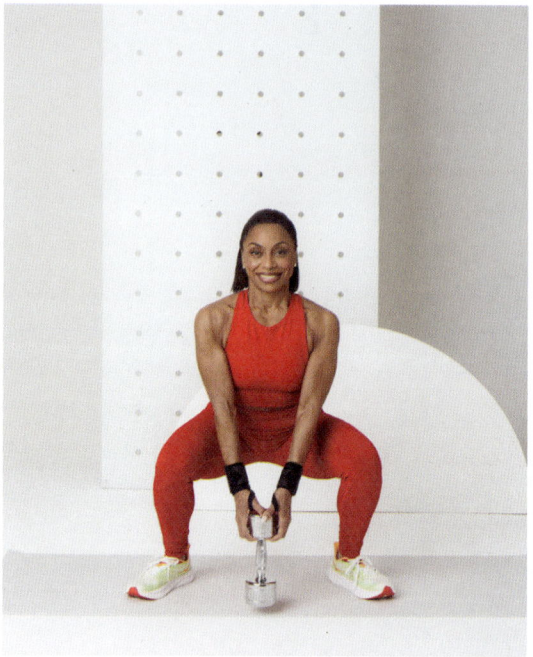

Dumbbell Sumo Squat

▶ Start standing with feet wider than hip-width apart, toes pointed out at 45 degrees, torso slightly forward, holding a dumbbell with both hands in front of you.

▶ Inhale, bend knees, and sink hips down until thighs are parallel to floor. Make sure to drive the knees outward.

▶ Exhale and drive through heels to return to starting position. That's 1 rep.

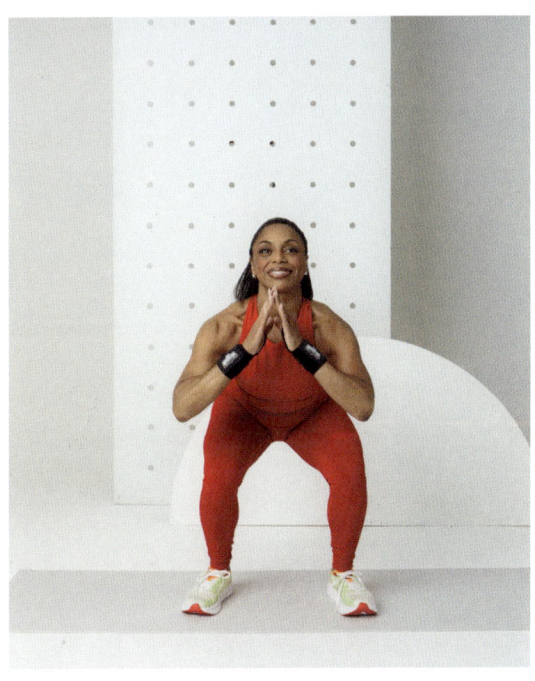

Jump Squat

▶ Stand with feet hip-width apart, toes slightly turned out, and arms by sides.

▶ Bend knees and sink hips to lower into a squat, then press through feet to explosively jump as high as you can into the air. Land softly on balls of feet and immediately lower into next squat. That's 1 rep; perform for prescribed number of reps or amount of time.

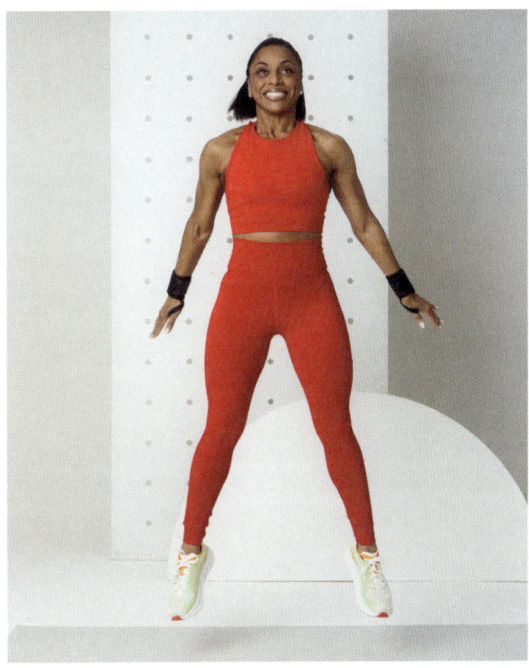

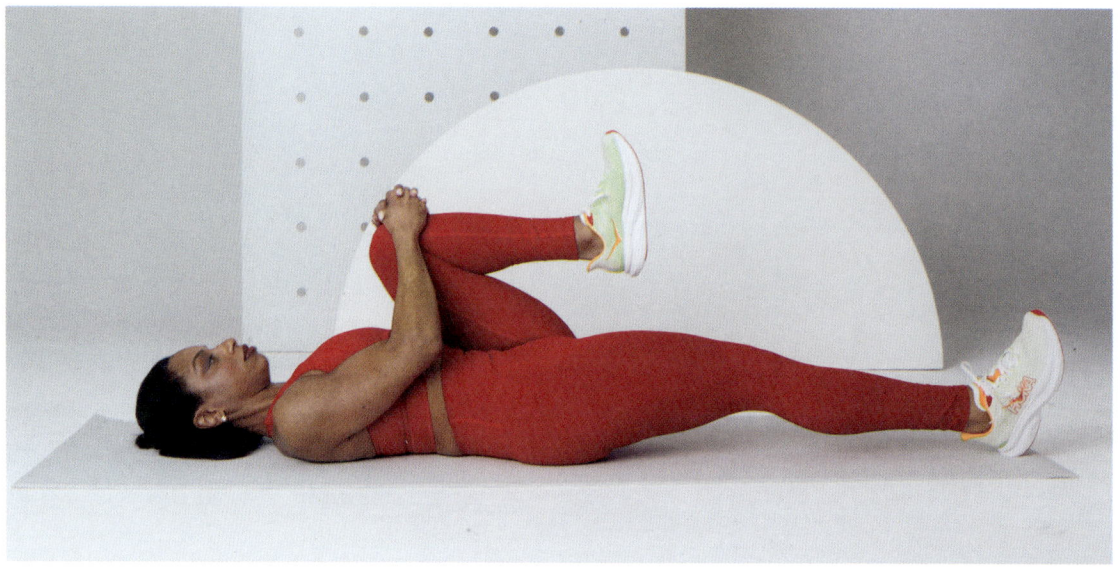

Lying Hip Flexor Stretch

▶ Lie faceup with legs fully extended and arms relaxed at sides, palms neutral.

▶ Take a deep breath, brace core, and push lower back into floor while slowly drawing one knee up toward your chest. As knee nears your chest, interlace fingers to latch hands over knee. Gently pull knee closer to chest.

▶ Hold for required time while keeping core tight and opposite leg fully extended. Slowly release knee and lower leg down to starting position.

Core

EXERCISE GUIDE Core

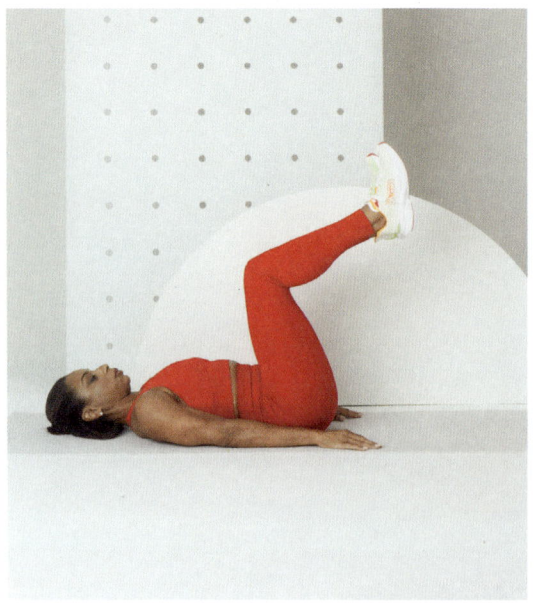
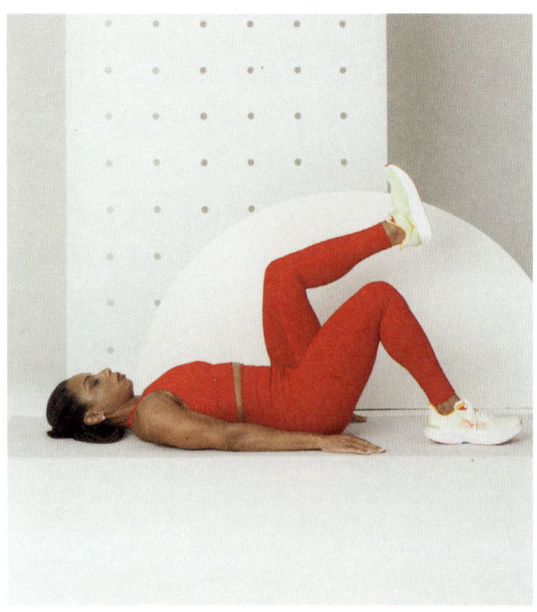
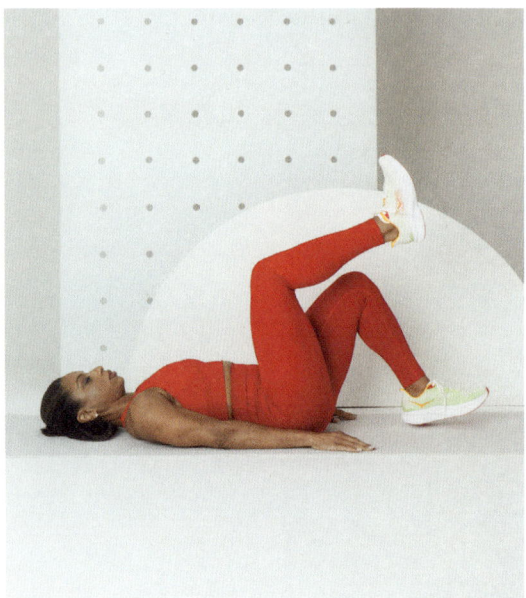

90/90 Tap

▶ Lie faceup with knees bent, feet flat on floor and hip-width apart.

▶ Exhale to squeeze and lift pelvic floor, drawing belly button toward spine. Engage core and keep knees bent as you raise one leg at a time until shins are parallel to floor.

▶ Slowly lower right foot to tap mat with heel, then reverse motion to return to start. Repeat with other leg. That's 1 rep.

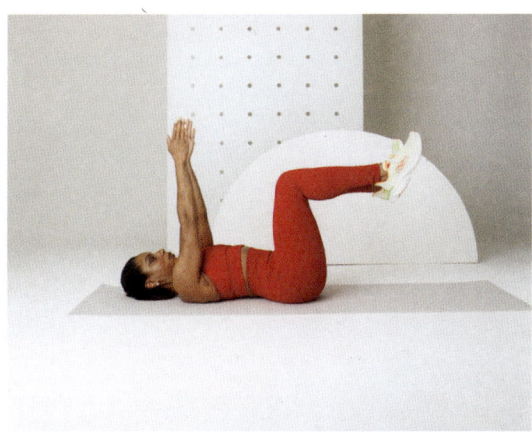

Deadbug

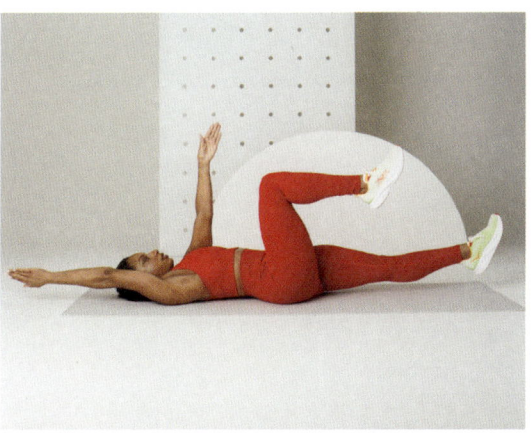

▶ Lie faceup on floor with arms extended over chest and legs bent 90 degrees (knees above hips).

▶ Keep lower back pressed to floor, brace core, then slowly and simultaneously extend and lower left leg until heel nearly touches floor and extend and lower right arm until hand nearly touches floor overhead. Pause, then return to start; that's 1 rep.

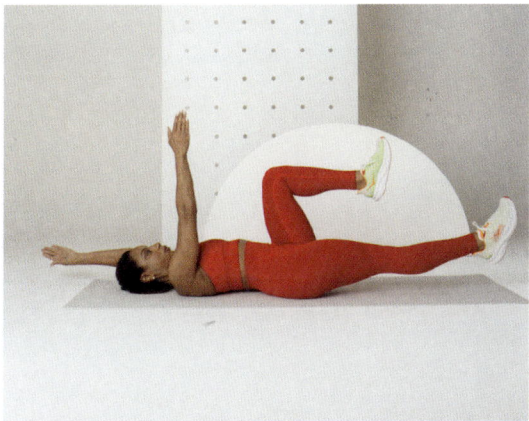

EXERCISE GUIDE Core

Loaded Deadbug

▶ Lie faceup on floor with arms extended over chest and legs bent 90 degrees (knees above hips), a light dumbbell in each hand.

▶ Keep lower back pressed to floor, brace core, then slowly and simultaneously extend and lower left leg until heel nearly touches floor and extend and lower right arm until hand nearly touches floor overhead. Pause, then return to start; that's 1 rep.

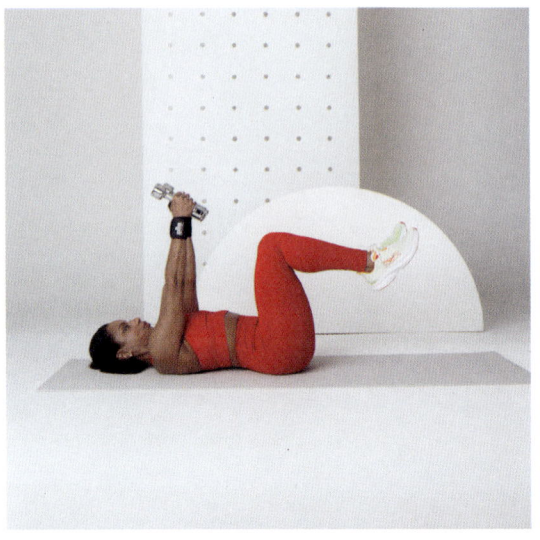

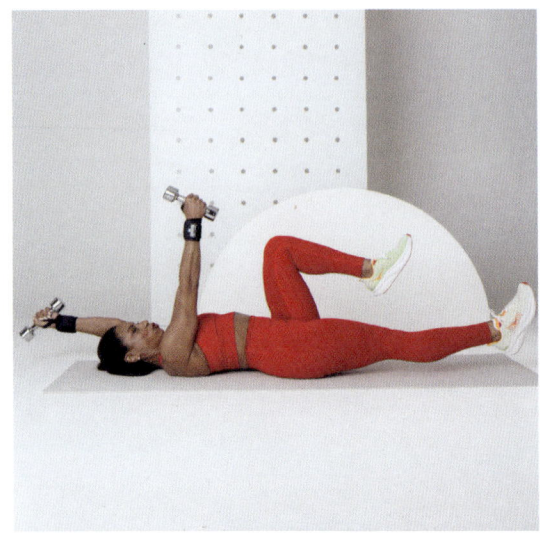

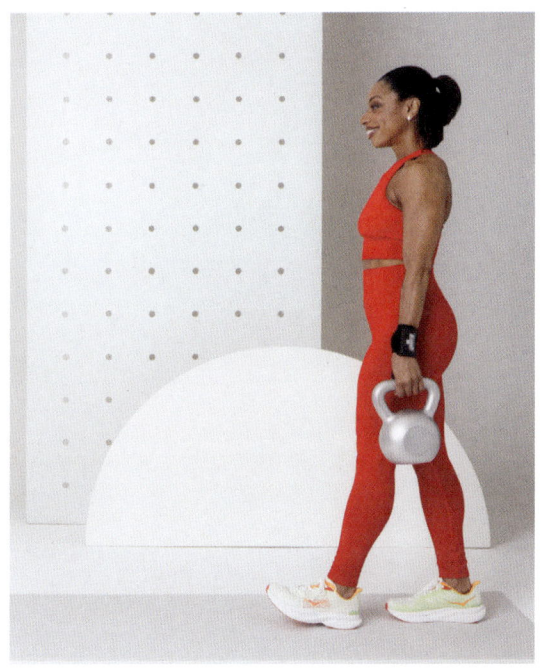 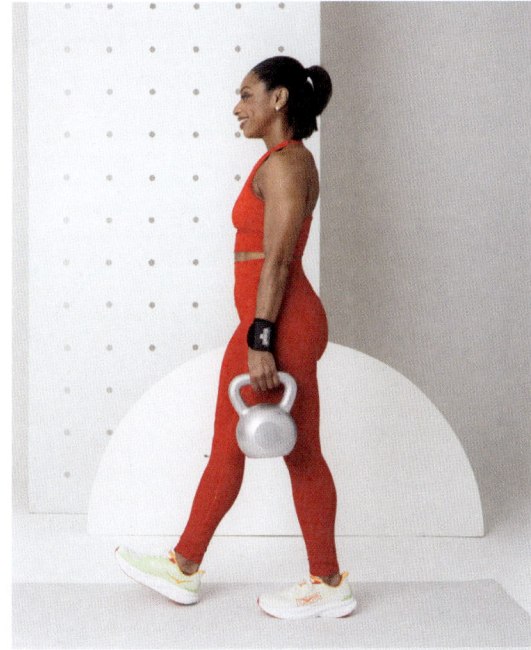

Farmer's Carry

- Stand up straight holding kettlebells or dumbbells at sides.
- Engage core and lift weights slightly out to sides, so they don't rest on legs. With control, take step forward with left foot. Repeat with right foot. Repeat for prescribed amount of steps.

EXERCISE GUIDE Core

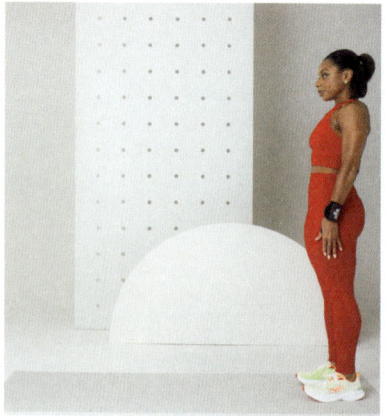
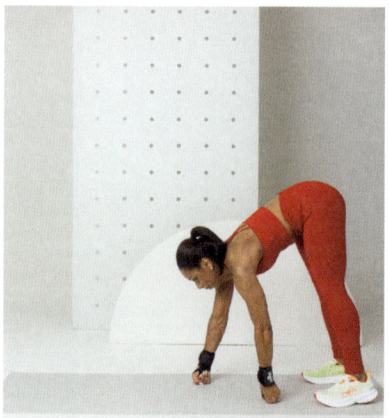
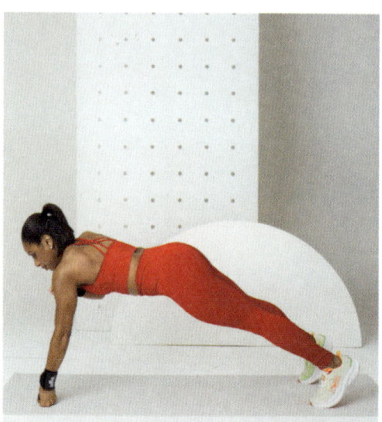
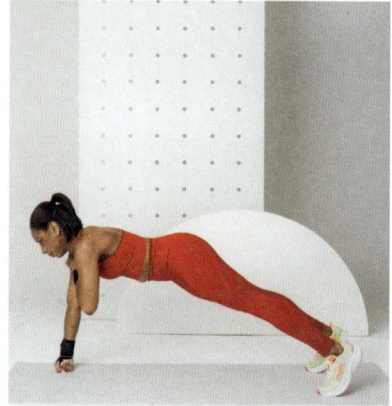

Inchworm Shoulder Tap

▶ Stand with feet hip-width apart. Reach down to floor and walk hands out into a plank position.

▶ Keeping hips square to floor, lift right hand to tap left shoulder. Return right hand to floor. Lift left hand to tap right shoulder. Return left hand to floor.

▶ Walk hands back to feet and return to standing. Perform for prescribed amount of time.

MODIFY IT: Performing this and other moves that require getting on your hands can put a lot of pressure on your wrists. Use your knuckles to alleviate the impact or put your palms flat on the floor if that's more comfortable.

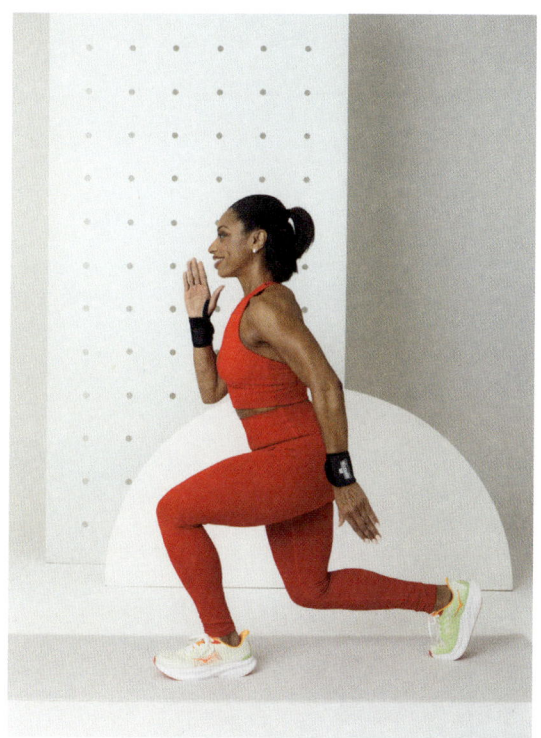 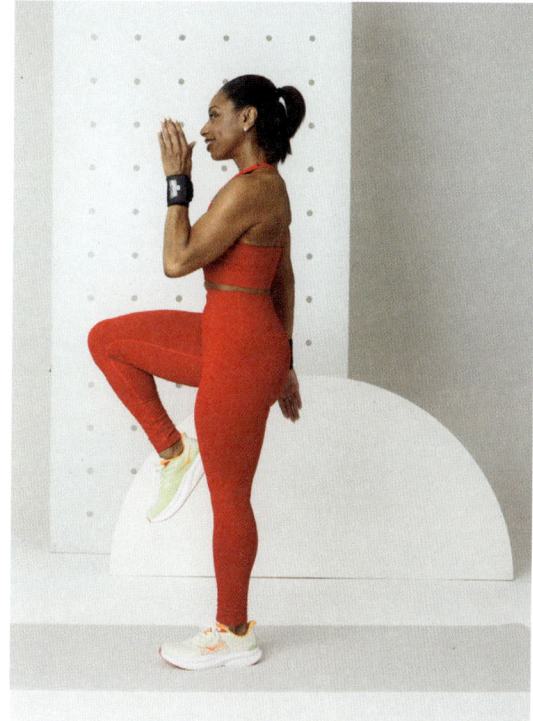

Knee Drive

▸ Stand with feet under hips. Step right foot a couple feet behind left foot.

▸ Bend back knee and drive it forward and up as high as you can. At the same time, swing arms with opposite leg, like you're running. Repeat on opposite side. Perform for prescribed amount of time.

EXERCISE GUIDE Core

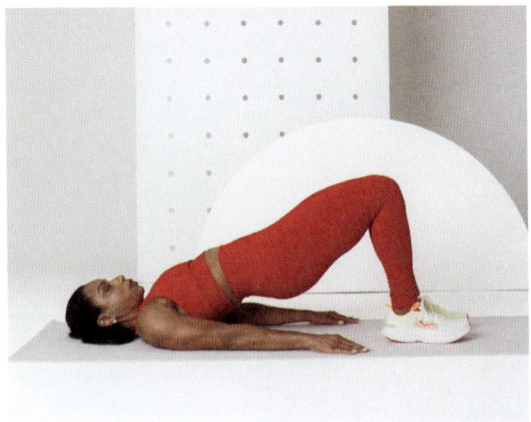

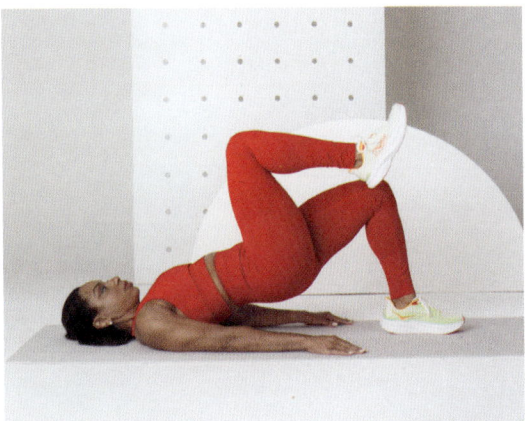

Marching Glute Bridge

▶ Lie faceup with knees bent and feet flat on floor.

▶ Squeeze glutes and lift hips off floor until body forms a straight line from knees to shoulders. Maintaining the hip position, raise right foot, knee bent at 90 degrees, until shin is parallel to floor. Lower it back to floor.

▶ Repeat on the left. Perform for prescribed amount of time.

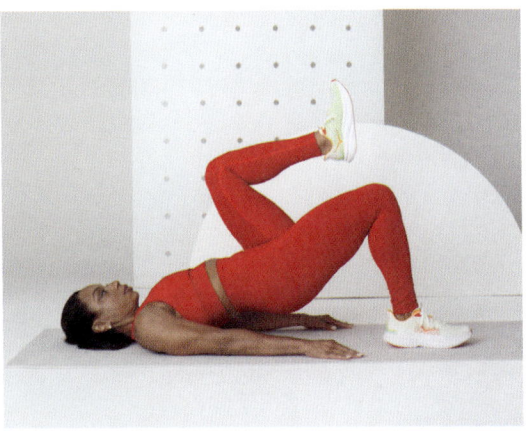

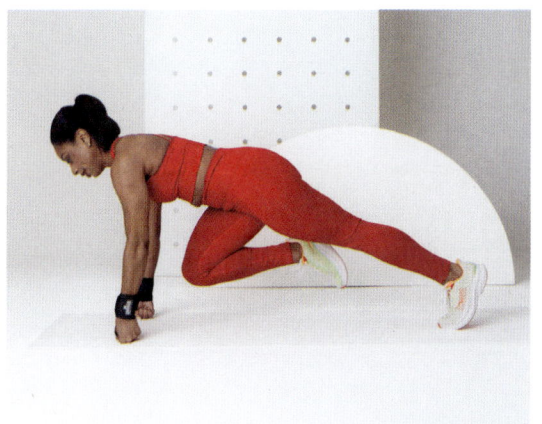
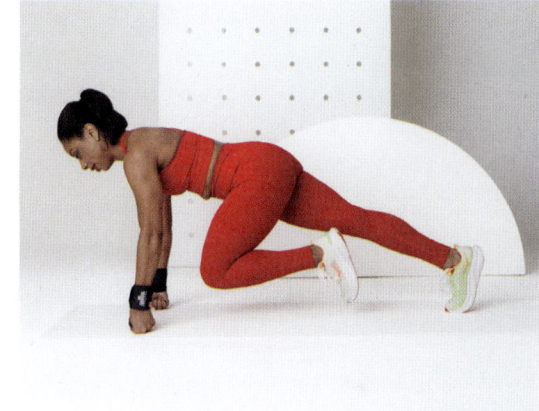

Mountain Climber

- Start in high plank, with shoulders over wrists, pelvis tucked, and ribs drawn toward hips.
- Drive right knee toward chest. Replace the right foot on mat and immediately repeat with left knee. That's 1 rep.

EXERCISE GUIDE Core

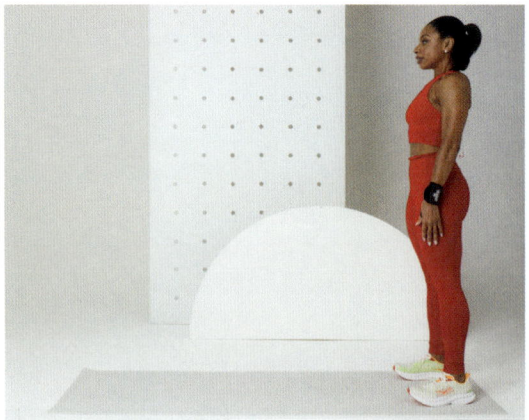

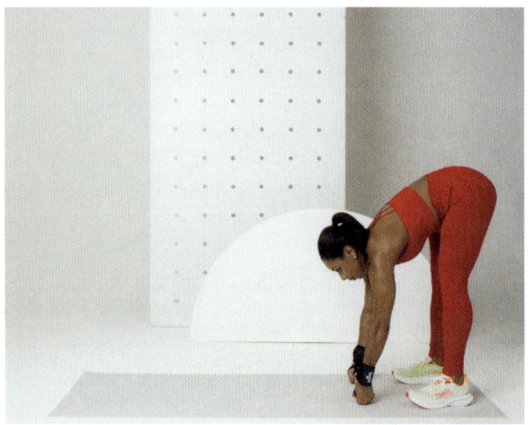

Plank Walkout

- Begin standing at back of mat with feet under hips and hands at sides.
- Fold forward at waist and bring hands to floor, then walk hands forward, stopping in high plank position with wrists under shoulders and legs extended straight.
- Reverse movement to return to start. That's 1 rep.

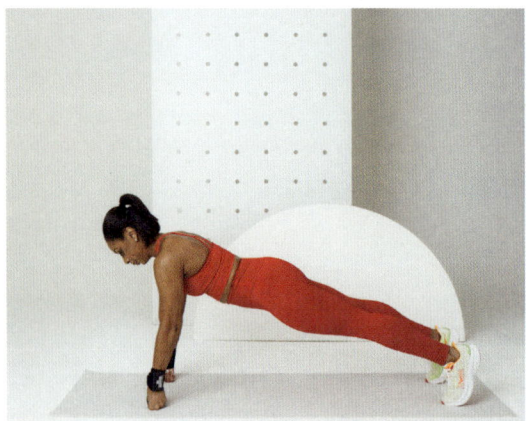

Reverse Crunch

- Lie faceup with arms by sides, legs extended, and feet lifted off floor, with toes pointed.
- Push down into arms and pull knees into chest until hips lift off floor.
- Slowly return to start. That's 1 rep.

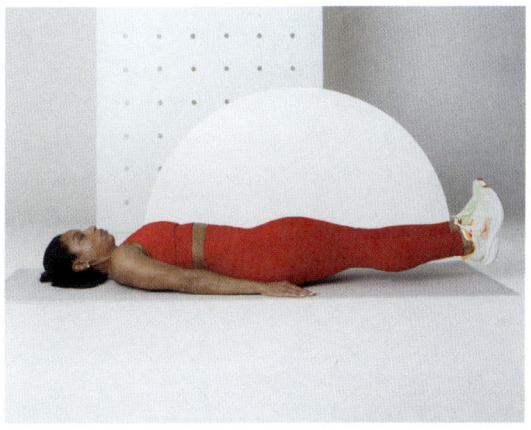

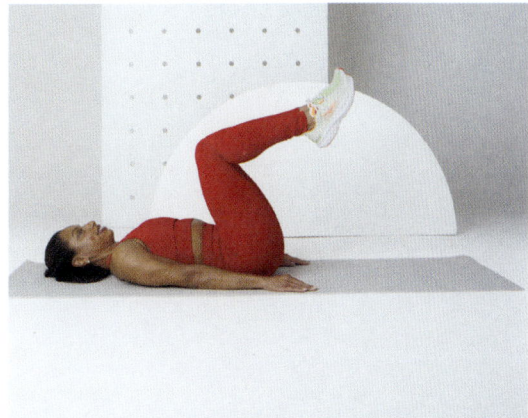

EXERCISE GUIDE Core

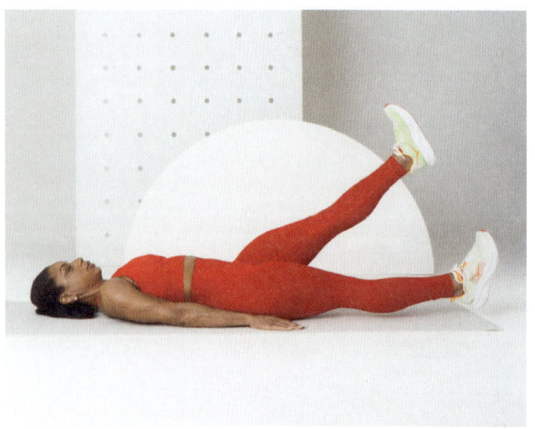 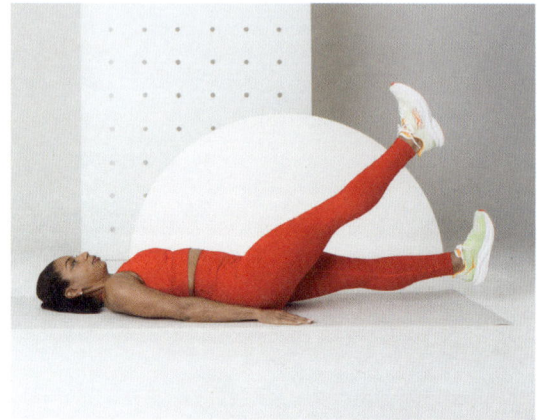

Scissor Kick

- Lie faceup with arms by sides, palms down, and elbows and lower back touching the floor.
- Engage core by pressing lower back into floor, tuck pelvis, and lift both legs about six inches off floor.
- Raise one leg to 45 degrees while maintaining the other leg about six inches off floor. Without letting feet touch floor, repeat with the opposite leg. That's 1 rep.

Superman

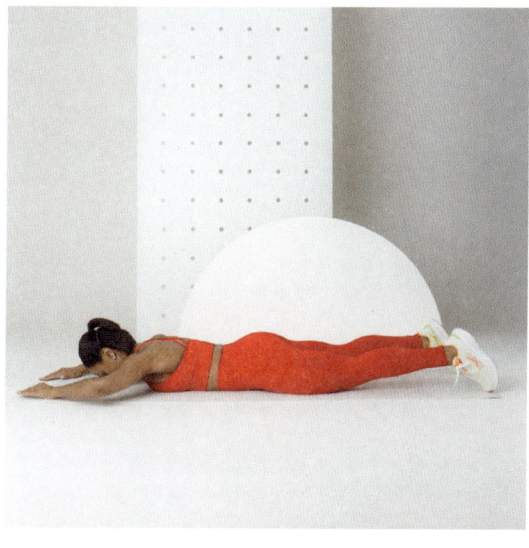

▶ Start lying facedown with arms and legs extended on floor so body forms one long line, forehead on mat.

▶ Engage abs, squeeze glutes, and lift all four limbs, plus chest and head a few inches off floor, keeping neck neutral by gazing at top of mat. Hold for three to five seconds, then slowly lower back to the starting position. That's 1 rep.

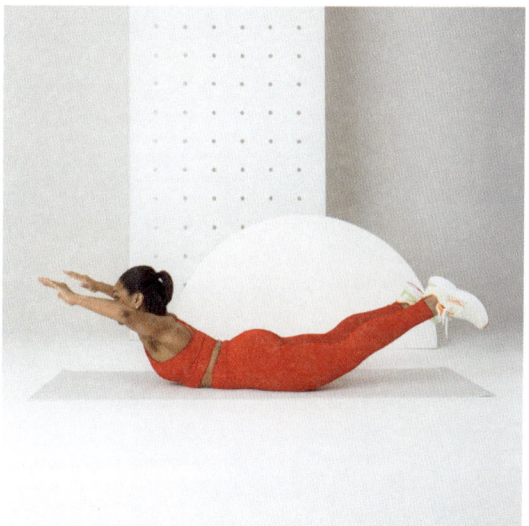

EXERCISE GUIDE Core

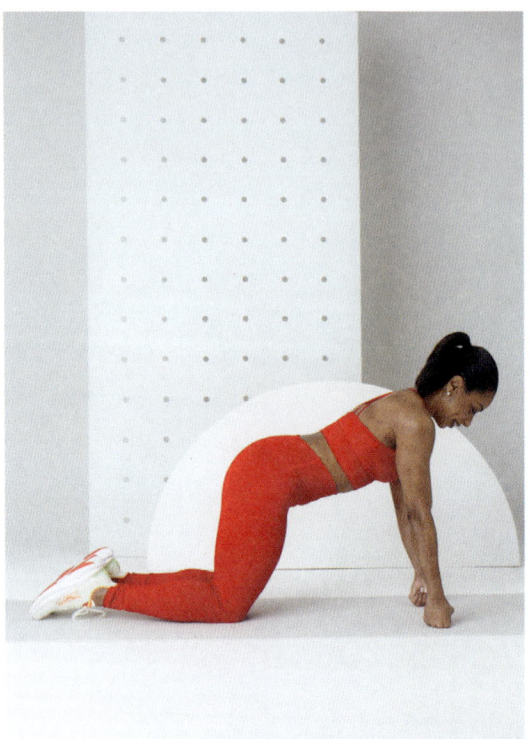
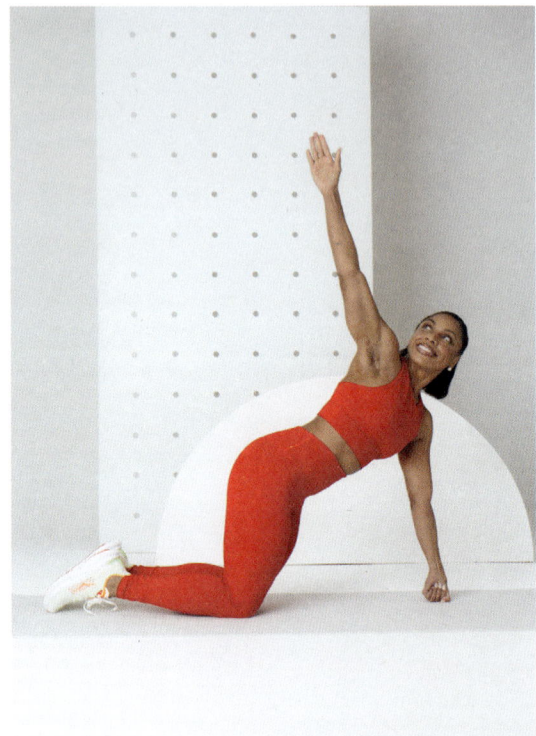

T-Spine Rotation

▶ Start in tabletop position with arms directly under shoulders and knees directly under hips.

▶ Keeping back straight, twist torso to right and lift right arm toward ceiling. Hold for prescribed amount of time, then return to start. Repeat with left arm.

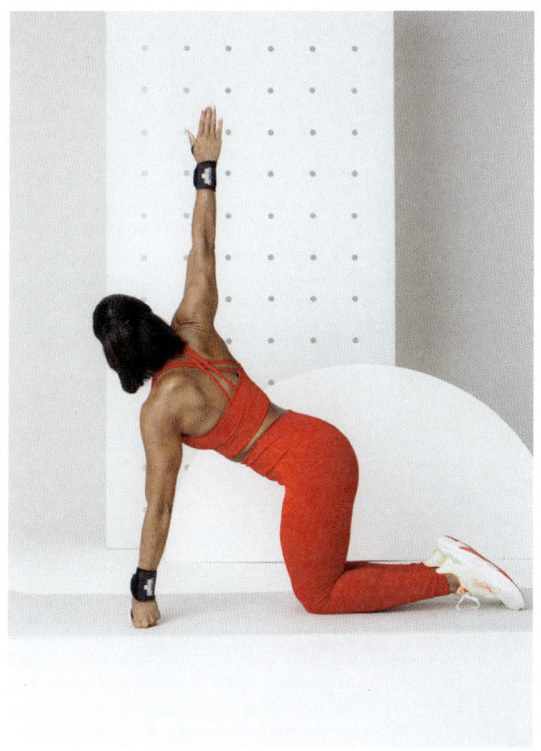 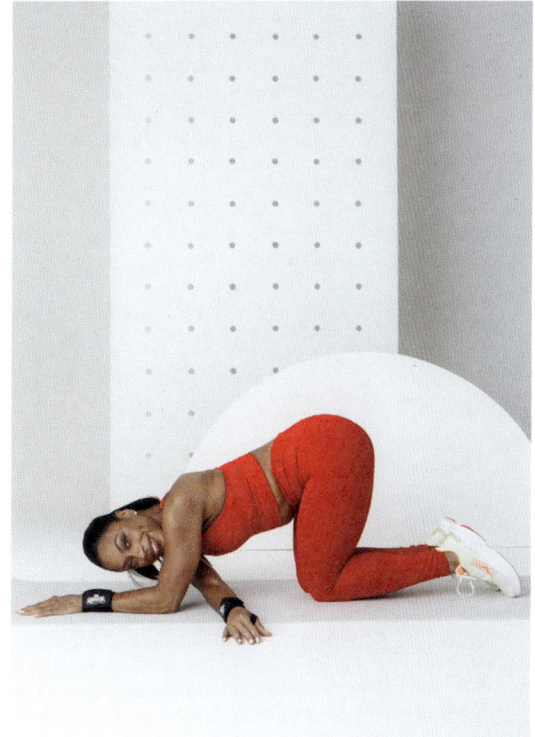

Thread the Needle

- Start in tabletop position with arms directly under shoulders and knees directly under hips.
- Lift right hand, arm straight toward the ceiling, then thread it under left shoulder so head can rest on floor facing left hand. Hold for prescribed amount of time. Imagine arm being gently pulled through to deepen stretch as upper back rotates. Repeat on left side.

EXERCISE GUIDE Core

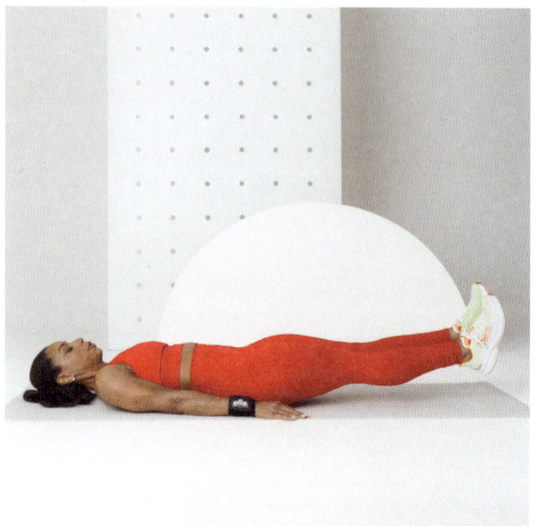

V-Up

▶ Start lying faceup with legs extended and arms by sides, both on mat. In one movement, lift upper body, arms, and legs, coming to balance on tailbone, forming a V shape with body, fingertips pointed toward toes.

▶ Lower back down. That's 1 rep.

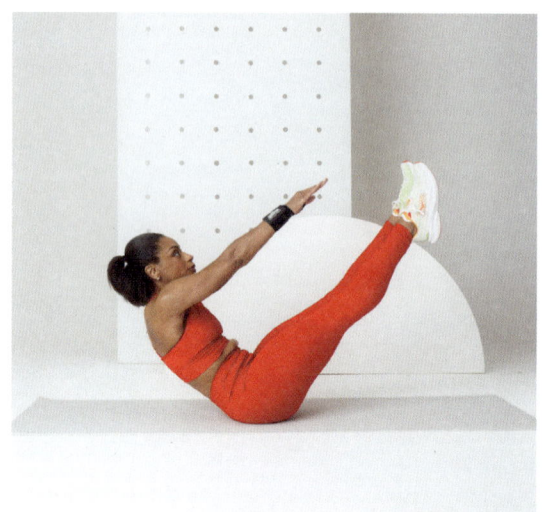

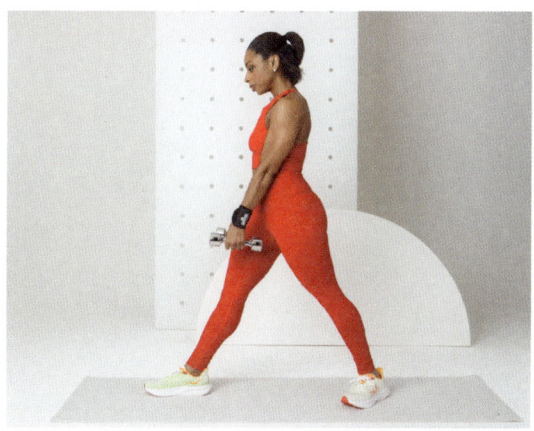

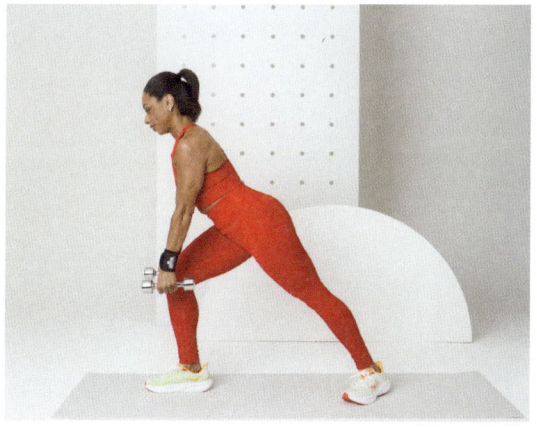

Warrior One Row

▶ Hold a pair of dumbbells at your sides, put left foot flat on floor about three feet behind your right foot, with toes pointed out, and bend right knee into a lunge.

▶ With your back flat, lower torso toward front knee, keeping arms straight.

▶ From this position, pull shoulder blades together and bend elbows to lift weights to sides of your chest. Slowly lower back to start. That's 1 rep.

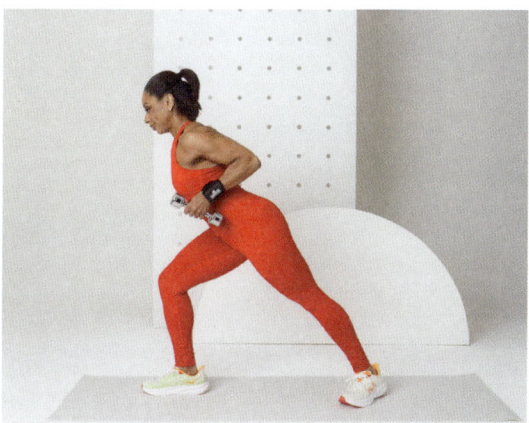

Total Body

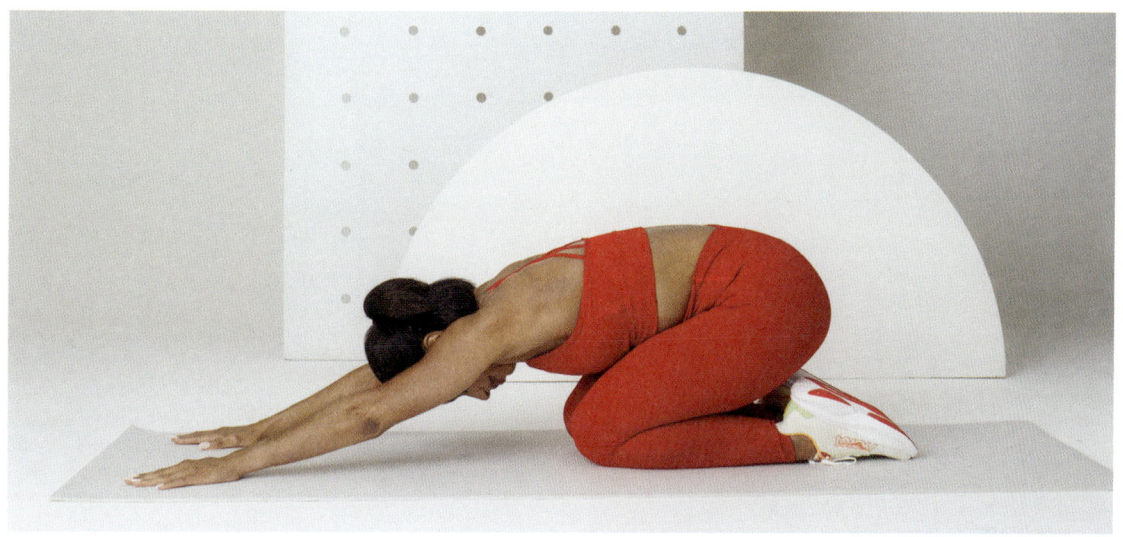

Child's Pose

- ▶ Start on all fours with hands under shoulders and knees wider than hips.
- ▶ Slowly sit hips back toward heels, and lean upper body forward, walking hands away from head until body forms a straight line from hips to hands. Rest forehead on mat and belly on thighs for prescribed amount of time.

EXERCISE GUIDE Total Body

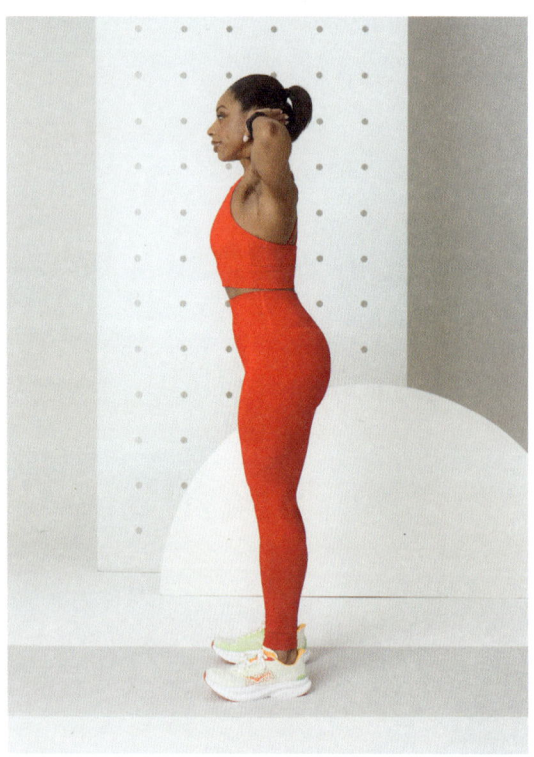
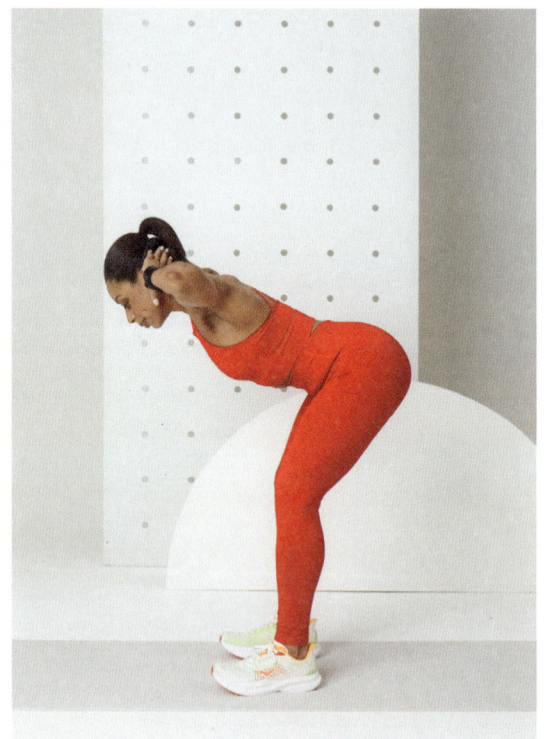

Good Morning

- Stand with knees slightly bent and hands behind head.
- Keeping back flat, hinge forward at hips, sending butt back. Bring hips forward and torso upright to stand up tall. That's 1 rep; perform for prescribed number of reps or amount of time.

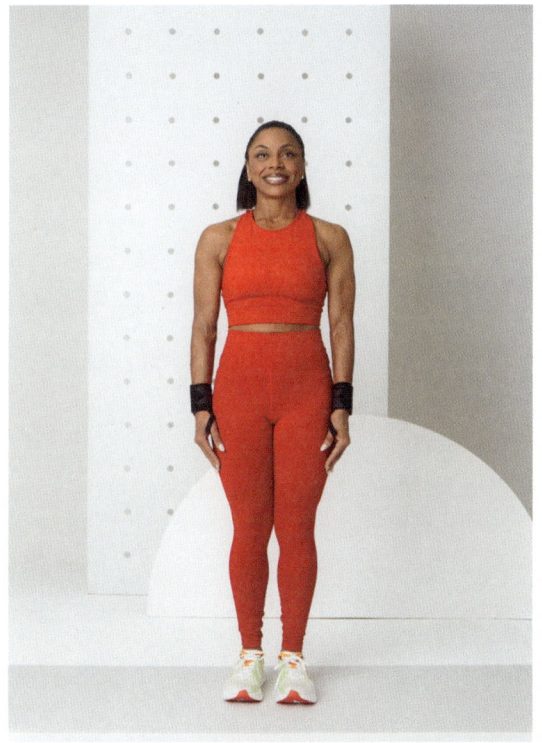 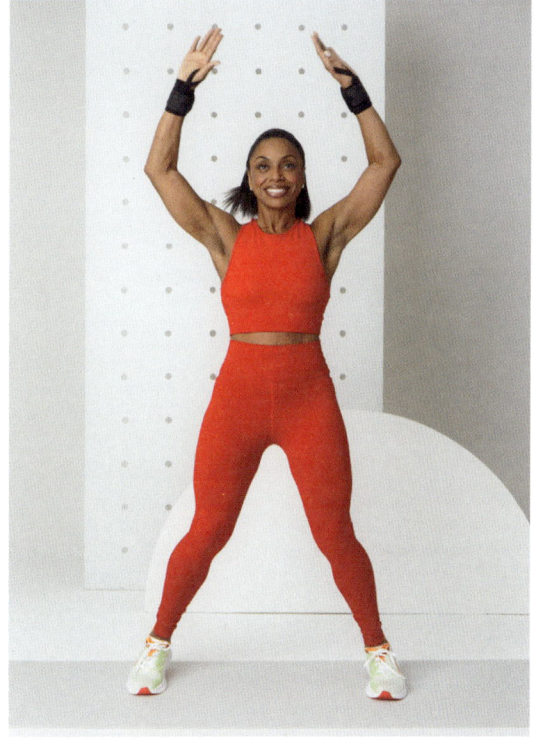

Jumping Jack

▶ Stand with feet together and arms at sides, then jump feet wider than shoulders as you lift arms overhead.

▶ Reverse move to return to start. Perform for prescribed amount of time.

EXERCISE GUIDE Total Body

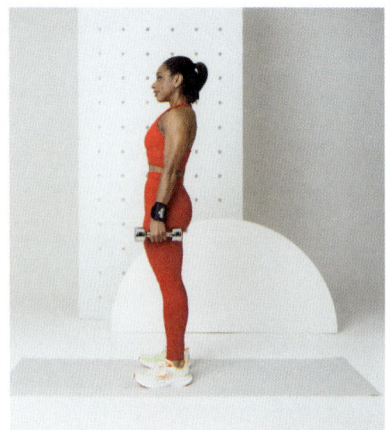
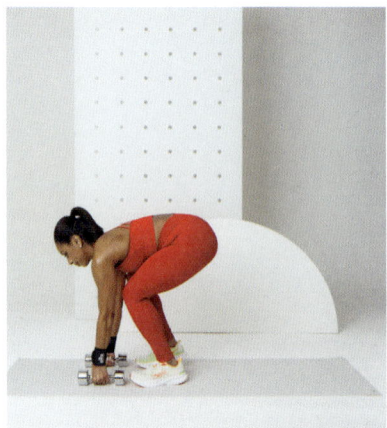
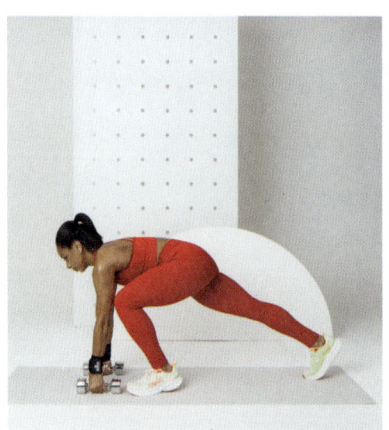
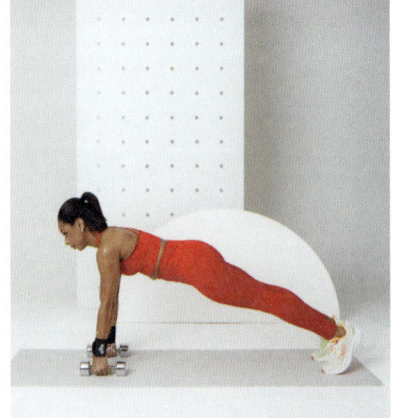

Modified Burpee

- ▶ Stand with feet slightly wider than hips, holding a dumbbell in each hand against sides, palms facing each other.
- ▶ Squat and place dumbbells on floor between feet. Keeping hands on dumbbells, walk back into plank position and hold.
- ▶ Reverse movement by walking back into squat, then stand. That's 1 rep.

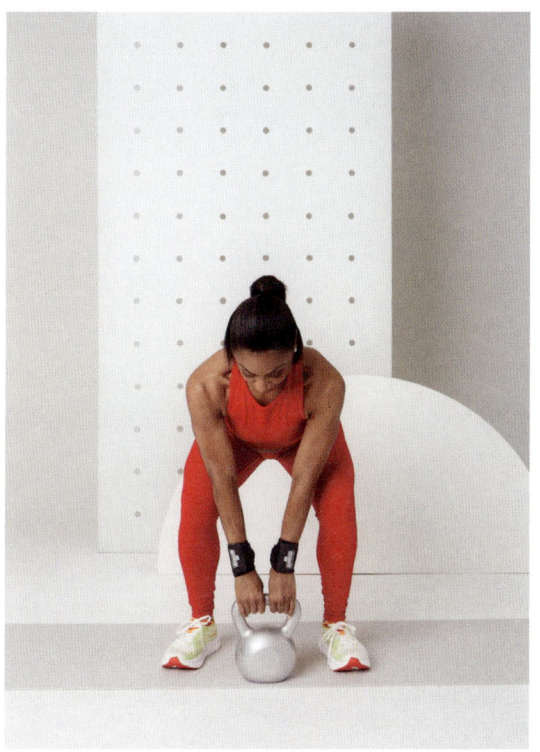 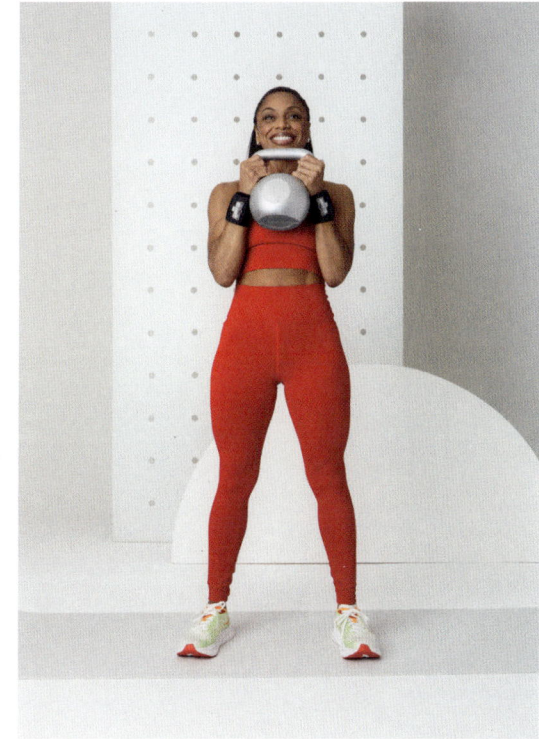

Dead Clean

▶ Stand with feet shoulder-width apart, kettlebell resting on floor below pelvis.

▶ Drop hips while keeping chest up, then grab bell horns with both hands. Activate lats by pretending you're holding something in both armpits.

▶ Press through feet to straighten through hips and drive bell up; hips should fully extend before bell reaches face height and you are in standing goblet position, elbows out in front of body.

▶ Reverse movement to return to start. That's 1 rep.

EXERCISE GUIDE Total Body

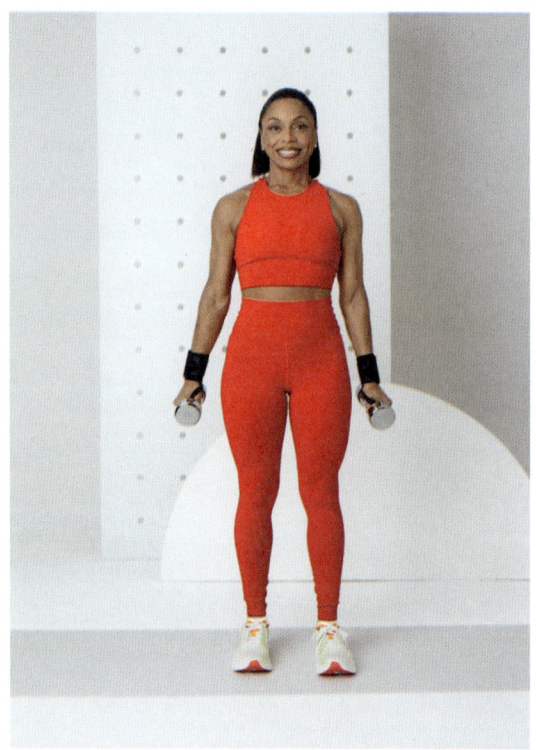 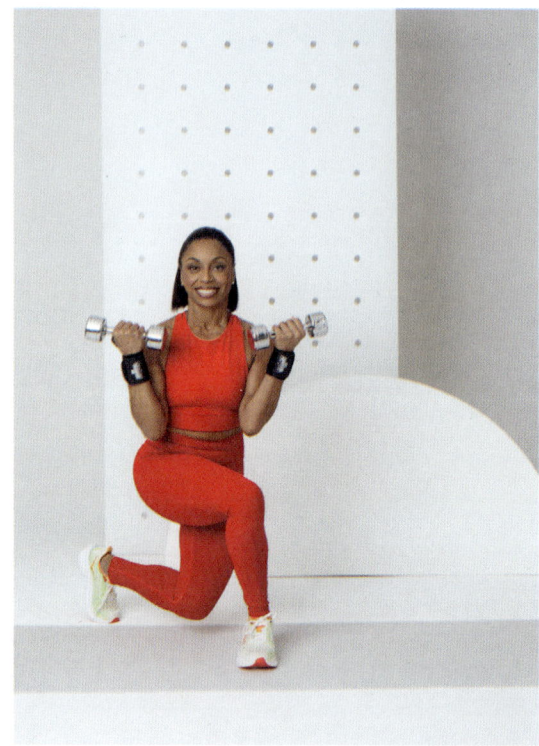

Curtsy Lunge With Biceps Curl

▶ Stand with feet hip-width apart, a dumbbell in each hand.

▶ Take a big step back with left leg, crossing it behind your right. Bend knees and lower hips until right thigh is nearly parallel to floor.

▶ At the same time, bend elbows and bring weights toward shoulders. Return to start. That's 1 rep.

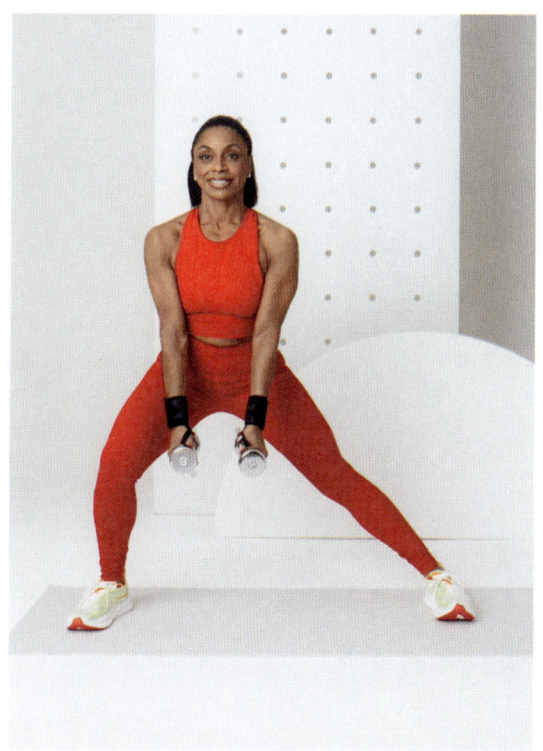
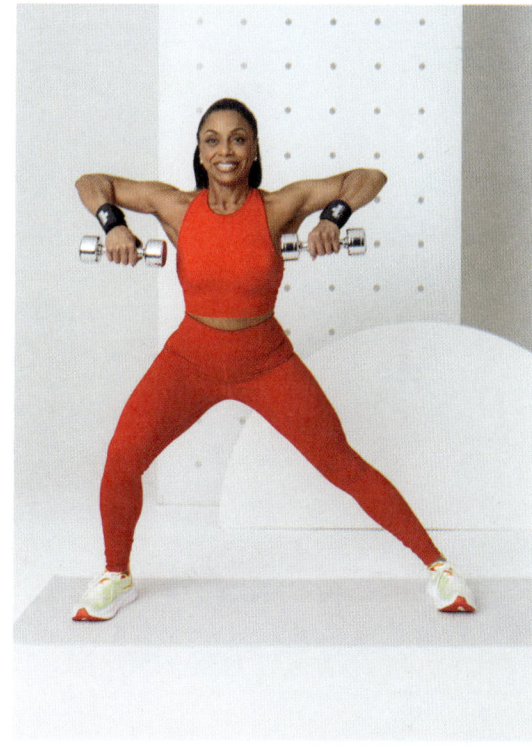

Side Lunge and Row

- Hold a pair of dumbbells at your sides and take a step to the right, lowering into a side lunge and moving weights toward floor, keeping your back flat.
- Bend elbows out to sides to raise dumbbells. Lower your arms and reverse movement to return to standing. That's 1 rep.

EXERCISE GUIDE Total Body

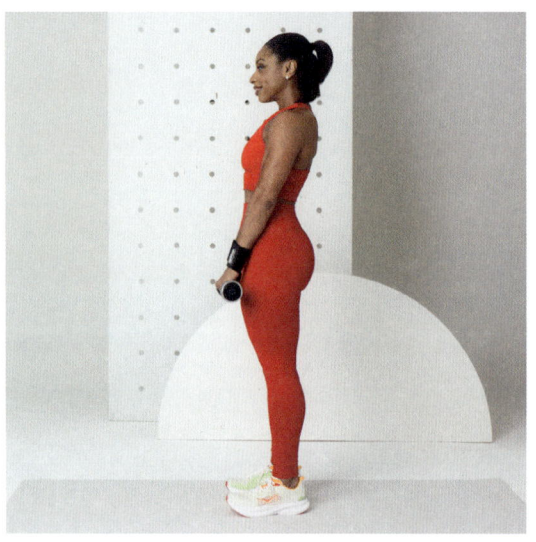
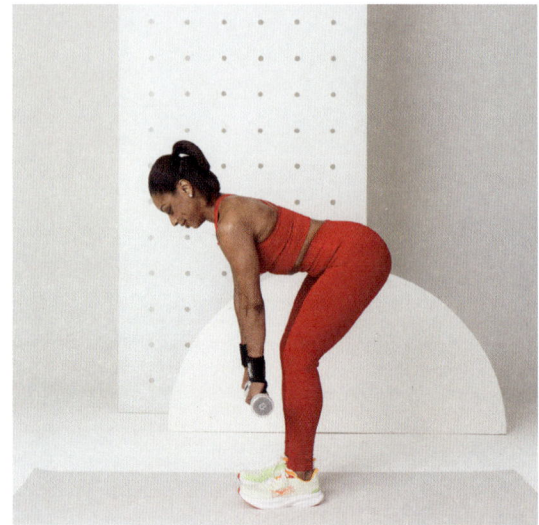

Deadlift and Row

▶ Stand with feet shoulder-width apart, a soft bend in knees, holding a dumbbell in each hand with palms facing legs and arms in front of thighs.

▶ Hinge hips as you lower dumbbells, keeping them close to thighs and shins. Pause at the bottom, then squeeze shoulder blades together and pull dumbbells toward rib cage.

▶ Reverse move by lowering dumbbells to shins, then driving through heels to stand with arms in front of thighs. That's 1 rep.

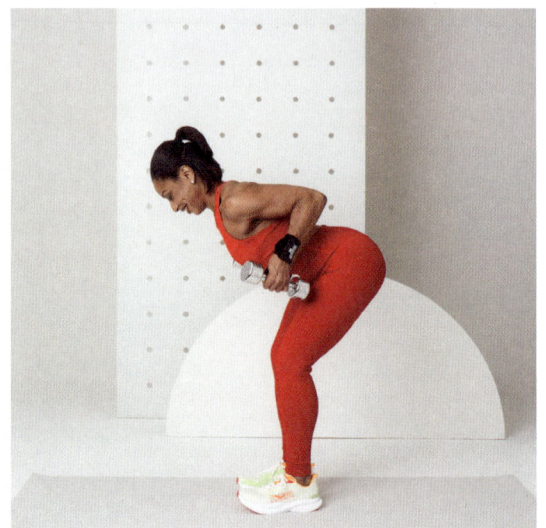

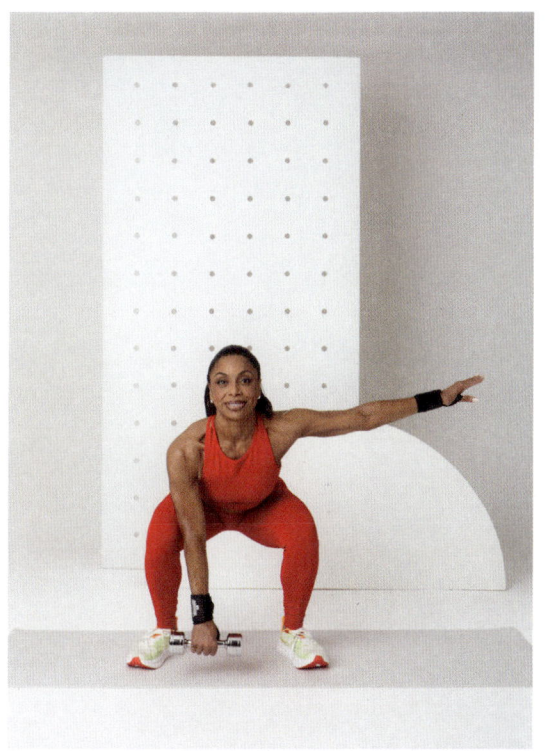
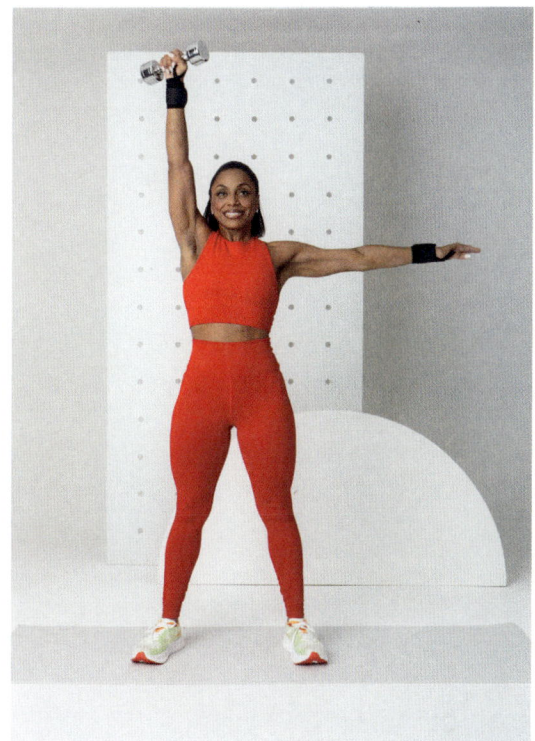

Squat and Snatch

▶ Start in a squat with a dumbbell between feet, holding it in one hand with an overhand grip.

▶ Power through hips, knees, and ankles to stand and accelerate dumbbell upward. Shrug shoulders and engage core to "flip" dumbbell, engaging lower body to support weight.

▶ Using lower body and core, extend dumbbell overhead with power. Reverse move to return to start. That's 1 rep.

EXERCISE GUIDE Total Body

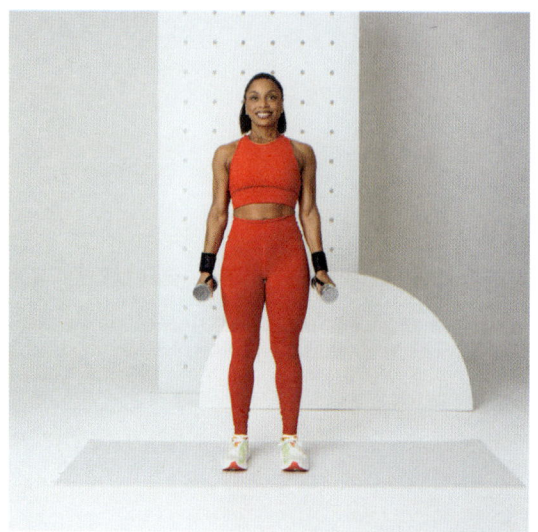
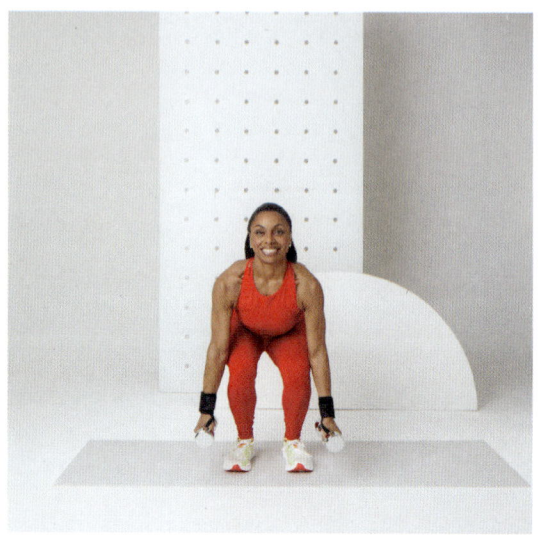
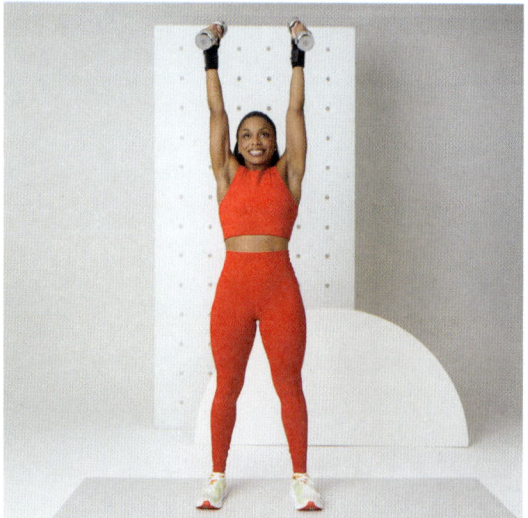

Squat to Overhead Press

▶ Start standing with feet shoulder-width apart holding a dumbbell in each hand, arms bent, elbows narrow, palms facing inward, and weights resting against sides.

▶ Inhale and lower body down into a squat. Engage core and, in one motion, exhale as you push through heels to stand and explosively press dumbbells overhead until arms are straight.

▶ Reverse movement to return to start. That's 1 rep.

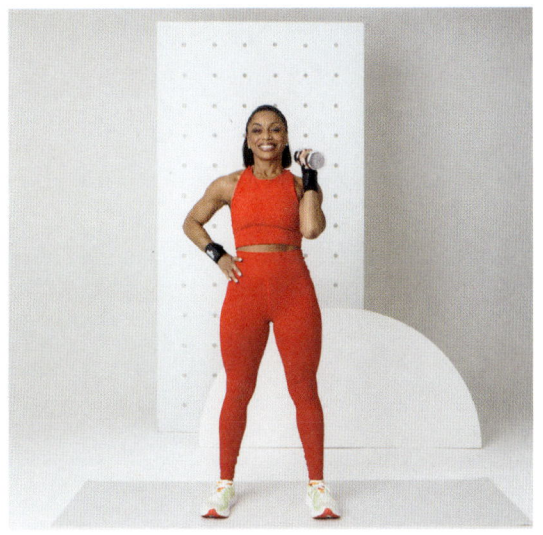

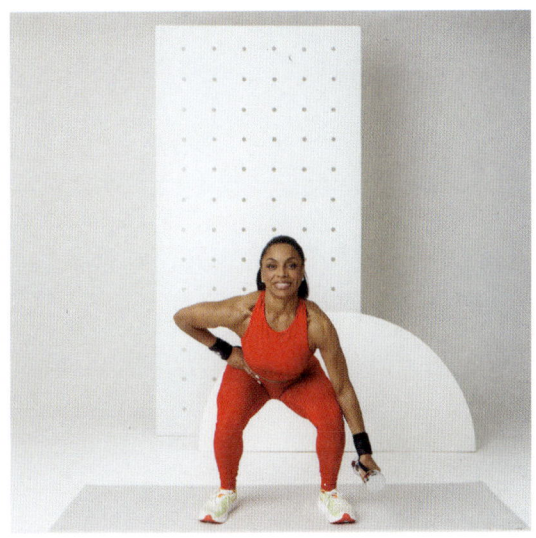

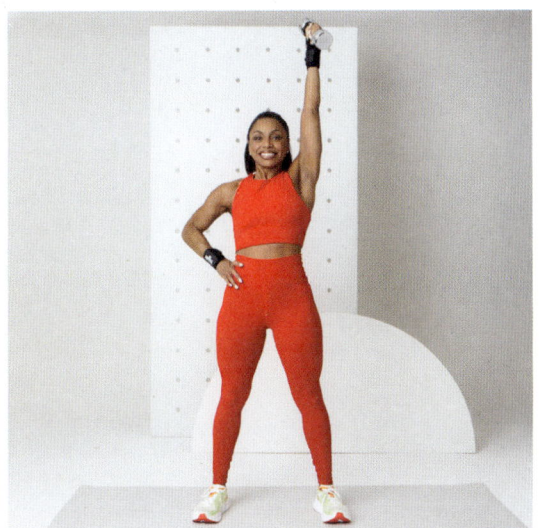

Squat to Single-Arm Overhead Press

▶ Stand with feet slightly wider than hips, holding a weight in left hand, with elbow bent so fist is in front of shoulder.

▶ Place right hand on right hip for balance, then push butt back while lowering into a squat until thighs are parallel to floor and extending arm with dumbbell down toward floor with control.

▶ Press through heels to stand and use the upward velocity to punch weight toward ceiling. That's 1 rep.

Notes:

Notes:

This book is intended as a reference volume only, not as medical advice. The information given here is designed to help you make informed decisions about your health. It is not intended as a substitute for medical or nutritional advice or any treatment that may have been prescribed by your doctor. If you suspect that you have a medical problem, we urge you to seek competent medical help.

© 2025 by Hearst Magazines, Inc.

All rights reserved. No part of this publication may be reproduced or transmitted in any form or by any means, electronic or mechanical, including photocopying, recording, or any other information storage and retrieval system, without the written permission of the publisher.

Women's Health® is a registered trademark of Hearst Magazines, Inc.

Photography by Eli Schmidt

Styling by Rose Lauture (Beach Riot top, Joja leggings, Mejuri earrings: cover, 13, 34; Beach Riot top, Joja leggings, Under Armour sneakers: 4; Beach Riot top, Mejuri earrings: 7, 60, 74; Beach Riot top, Beyond Yoga shorts, Reebok sneakers: 8-9, 14; Nike sports bra, Fanka jacket, Mejuri earrings: 16-17; Nike sports bra, Alo Yoga shorts, Fanka jacket, Mejuri earrings: 19, 21, 23; Beach Riot top and leggings, Hoka sneakers, Mejuri earrings: 24, 36-44, 48-58, 62-72, 76-86, 91-139; Beach Riot jumpsuit, Under Armour sneakers, Mejuri earrings: 28-30; Beach Riot top, Mejuri earrings: 46; Beach Riot top, Beyond Yoga shorts, Mejuri earrings: 89; Beach Riot jumpsuit, Mejuri earrings: back cover)

Hair by Anike Rabiu

Makeup by Magdalena Major

Book design by Caroline Pickering

Library of Congress Cataloging-in-Publication Data is on file with the publisher.

ISBN 978-1-955710-40-4

Printed in China

2 4 6 8 10 9 7 5 3 1 hardcover

HEARST

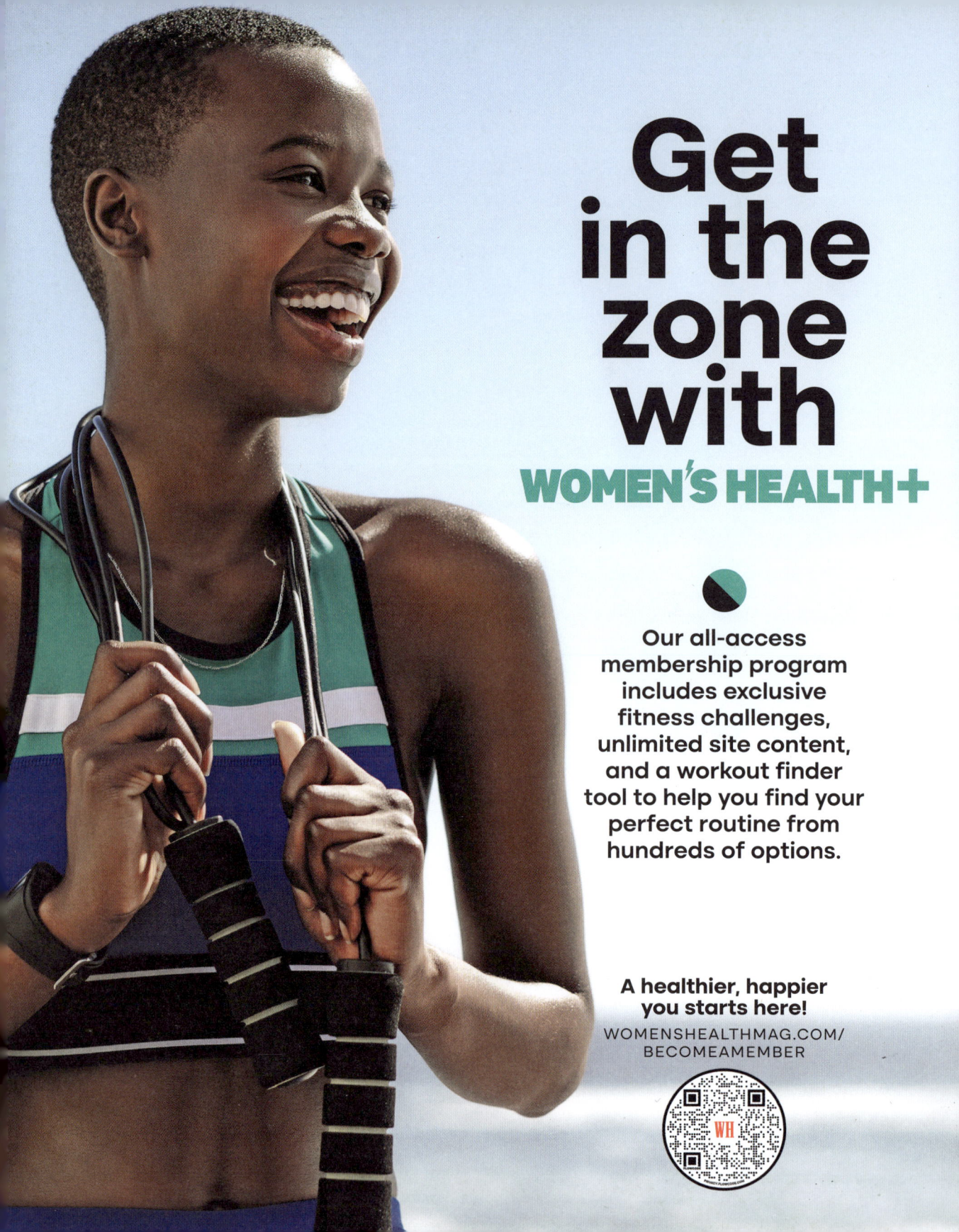